Temporomandibular Disorders: the Current Perspective

Editors

DAVIS C. THOMAS
STEVEN R. SINGER

DENTAL CLINICS OF NORTH AMERICA

www.dental.theclinics.com

April 2023 • Volume 67 • Number 2

ELSEVIER

1600 John F. Kennedy Boulevard ● Suite 1800 ● Philadelphia, Pennsylvania, 19103-2899

http://www.dental.theclinics.com

DENTAL CLINICS OF NORTH AMERICA Volume 67, Number 2
April 2023 ISSN 0011-8532, ISBN: 978-0-323-93985-0

Editor: John Vassallo; j.vassallo@elsevier.com
Developmental Editor: Ann Gielou M. Posedio

Dental Clinics of North America (ISSN 0011-8532) is published quarterly by Elsevier Inc., 360 Park Avenue South, New York, NY 10010-1710. Months of issue are January, April, July, and October. Business and Editorial Offices: 1600 John F. Kennedy Boulevard, Suite 1800, Philadelphia, PA 19103-2899. Periodicals postage paid at New York, NY and additional mailing offices. Subscription prices are $333.00 per year (domestic individuals), $692.00 per year (domestic institutions), $100.00 per year (domestic students/residents), $388.00 per year (Canadian individuals), $897.00 per year (Canadian institutions), $100.00 per year (Canadian students/residents) $454.00 per year (international individuals), $897.00 per year (international institutions), and $200.00 per year (international students/residents). International air speed delivery is included in all *Clinics* subscription prices. All prices are subject to change without notice. **POSTMASTER:** Send address changes to *Dental Clinics of North America*, Elsevier Health Sciences Division, Subscription Customer Service, 3251 Riverport Lane, Maryland Heights, MO 63043. **Customer Service (orders, claims, online, change of address): Elsevier Health Sciences Division, Subscription Customer Service, 3251 Riverport Lane, Maryland Heights, MO 63043. Tel: 1-800-654-2452 (U.S. and Canada). Fax: 314-447-8029. E-mail: journalscustomerservice-usa@elsevier.com (for print support); journalsonlinesupport-usa@elsevier. com (for online support).**

Reprints. For copies of 100 or more, of articles in this publication, please contact the Commercial Reprints Department, Elsevier Inc., 360 Park Avenue South, New York, NY 10010-1710. Tel.: 212-633-3874; Fax: 212-633-3820; E-mail: reprints@elsevier.com.

The Dental Clinics of North America is covered in *MEDLINE/PubMed (Index Medicus), Current Contents/Clinical Medicine, ISI/BIOMED* and *Clinahl.*

Contributors

EDITORS

DAVIS C. THOMAS, BDS, DDS, MSD, MSc Med, MSc
Clinical Associate Professor, Program Director, Preceptorship in General Dentistry, Department of Diagnostic Sciences, Rutgers School of Dental Medicine, Newark, New Jersey, USA

STEVEN R. SINGER, DDS
Professor and Chair, Department of Diagnostic Sciences, Interim Director, Division of Oral and Maxillofacial Radiology, Rutgers School of Dental Medicine, Newark, New Jersey, USA

AUTHORS

JESSICA AILANI, MD, FAHS
Director, Georgetown Headache Center, Professor of Clinical Neurology, Vice Co-Chair Strategic Planning Neurology, MedStar Georgetown University Hospital, Washington, DC, USA

SOWMYA ANANTHAN, BDS, DMD, MSD
Department of Diagnostic Sciences, Associate Professor, Center for Temporomandibular Disorders and Orofacial Pain, Rutgers School of Dental Medicine, Newark, New Jersey, USA

STEVEN D. BENDER, DDS
Department of Oral and Maxillofacial Surgery, Clinical Associate Professor, College of Dentistry, Texas A&M Health, Dallas, Texas, USA

THOMAS BORNHARDT, DDS, MSC
Assistant Professor, Department of Integral Adult Care Dentistry, Temporomandibular Disorder, Orofacial Pain Program, Sleep and Pain Research Group, Faculty of Dentistry, Universidad de La Frontera, Temuco, Chile

DAVID BRISS, DMD
Associate Professor, Department of Orthodontics, Rutgers School of Dental Medicine, Newark, New Jersey, USA

ELI ELIAV, DMD, MSc, PhD
Professor and Director, Eastman Institute for Oral Health, University of Rochester Medical Center, Rochester, New York, USA

MAHNAZ FATAHZADEH, DMD, MSD
Professor, Division of Oral Medicine, Department of Oral Medicine, Rutgers School of Dental Medicine, Newark, New Jersy, USA

ANTONIO ROMERO GARCIA, DDS, PhD, MSc
CranioClinic, Valencia and Dental Sleep Solutions, Valencia, Spain

JEAN-PAUL GOULET, DDS, MSD, FRCD
Professeur Émérite, Spécialiste en médecine buccale, Faculté de médecine dentaire, Pavillon de Médecine Dentaire, Université Laval, Québec, Canada

PETER HENEIN, DMD
Oral and Maxillofacial Surgery Resident, Rutgers School of Dental Medicine

VERONICA ITURRIAGA, DDS, MSC, PhD
Assistant Professor, Department of Integral Adult Care Dentistry, Temporomandibular Disorder, Orofacial Pain Program, Sleep and Pain Research Group, Faculty of Dentistry, Universidad de La Frontera, Temuco, Chile

SHANKAR IYER, DDS, MDS
Private Practice limited to Prosthodontics, Elizabeth, New Jersey, USA; Assistant Clinical Professor, Departments of Prosthodontics and Periodontics, Rutgers University, Newark, New Jersey, USA

MYTHILI KALLADKA, BDS, MSD
Assistant Professor, Eastman Institute for Oral Health, Rochester, New York, USA

JUNAD KHAN, DDS, MSD, MPH, PhD
Associate Professor and Program Director, Department of Orofacial Pain and Temporomandibular Disorders, Eastman Institute for Oral Health, Rochester, New York, USA

GARY D. KLASSER, DMD
Cert. Orofacial Pain, Professor, Department of Diagnostic Sciences, School of Dentistry, Louisiana State University Health Sciences Center, New Orleans, Los Angeles, USA

FRANK LOBBEZOO, DDS, PhD
Professor and Head, Department of Orofacial Pain and Dysfunction, Academic Centre for Dentistry Amsterdam (ACTA), University of Amsterdam and Vrije Universiteit Amsterdam, Amsterdam, the Netherlands

DANIELE MANFREDINI, DDS, PhD
Professor and Head, Facial Pain Unit, Department of Biomedical Technologies, School of Dentistry, University of Siena, Viale Bracci, Siena, Italy

STANLEY MARKMAN, DDS
Clinical Assistant Professor, Department of Diagnostic Sciences, Rutgers School of Dental Medicine, Newark, New Jersey, USA

ISABEL MORENO-HAY, DDS PhD ABOP ABDSM
Division Chief and Program Director, Orofacial Pain, Assistant Professor, College of Dentistry, University of Kentucky, Kentucky Clinic, Lexington, Kentucky, USA

MEL MUPPARAPU, DMD, MDS, Dipl ABOMR
Professor of Oral Medicine, Director of Radiology, University of Pennsylvania School of Dental Medicine, Philadelphia, Pennsylvania, USA

CIBELE NASRI-HEIR, DDS, MSD
Department of Diagnostic Sciences, Associate Professor, Center for Temporomandibular Disorders and Orofacial Pain, Rutgers School of Dental Medicine, The State University, Newark, New Jersey, USA

RICHARD A. PERTES, DDS
Department of Diagnostic Sciences, Clinical Professor, Center for Temporomandibular Disorders and Orofacial Pain, Rutgers School of Dental Medicine, Newark, New Jersey, USA

SAMUEL Y. P. QUEK, DMD, MPH
Professor, Department of Diagnostic Sciences, Rutgers School of Dental Medicine, Newark, New Jersey, USA

PAUL EMILE ROSSOUW, MChD, PhD
Professor and Chair, Department of Orthodontics and Dentofacial Orthopedics, Eastman Institute for Oral Health, University of Rochester, Rochester, New York, USA

STEVEN R. SINGER, DDS
Professor and Chair, Department of Diagnostic Sciences, Interim Director, Division of Oral and Maxillofacial Radiology, Rutgers School of Dental Medicine, Newark, New Jersey, USA

GAYATHRI SUBRAMANIAN, BDS, PhD, DMD
Associate Professor, Department of Diagnostic Sciences, Rutgers School of Dental Medicine, Newark, New Jersey, USA

NARUTHORN TANAIUTCHAWOOT, DMD, MSD
Rutgers School of Dental Medicine, Newark, New Jersey, USA

DAVIS C. THOMAS, BDS, DDS, MSD, MSc Med, MSc
Clinical Associate Professor, Program Director, Preceptorship in General Dentistry, Department of Diagnostic Sciences, Rutgers School of Dental Medicine, Newark, New Jersey, USA

RIVA TOUGER-DECKER, PhD, RD, CDN, FADA
Professor, Department of Diagnostic Sciences, Rutgers School of Dental Medicine, Professor and Associate Dean of Global Affairs, Rutgers School of Health Professions, Newark, New Jersey, USA

NICOL VELASQUEZ, DDS
Temporomandibular Disorder, Orofacial Pain Program, Faculty of Dentistry, Universidad de La Frontera, Temuco, Chile

ANDREW YOUNG, DDS, MSD
Assistant Professor, Arthur A. Dugoni School of Dentistry, University of the Pacific, San Francisco, California, USA

VINCENT B. ZICCARDI, DDS, MD, FACS
Department of Oral and Maxillofacial Surgery, Professor, Chair and Residency Director, Associate Dean of Hospital Affairs, Rutgers School of Dental Medicine, Newark, New Jersey, USA

JULYANA GOMES ZAGURY, DMD, MSD
Adjunct Assistant Professor, Department of Diagnostic Sciences, Rutgers School of Dental Medicine, Newark, New Jersey, USA

Contents

Temporomandibular Joint: Review of Anatomy and Clinical Implications   199

Veronica Iturriaga, Thomas Bornhardt, and Nicol Velasquez

> Temporomandibular joints (TMJ) are one of the most complex joints. Each
> one is located on one side of the face, and are composed of mandibular
> fossa, joint tubercle, and condylar process of mandible, separated by an
> articular disk. To these structures are attached ligaments and muscles,
> which will provide stability and movement. When TMJs work properly,
> jaw movements can be performed without pain or discomfort. It is impor-
> tant to mention that the complex formed by both TMJs will confront the
> maxillary with the mandibular bone and therefore will be related to the oc-
> clusion, linking these structures during growth and development.

**Classification and Diagnosis of Temporomandibular Disorders and
Temporomandibular Disorder Pain**   211

Gary D. Klasser, Jean-Paul Goulet, and Isabel Moreno-Hay

> Designing classification systems and developing diagnostic criteria for
> temporomandibular disorders is difficult. An appreciation of the utility
> and applicability of these entities requires an understanding of the impor-
> tance of each, the differences between the two, and how they may be opti-
> mally operationalized for both clinical and research activities in light of their
> inherent advantages and limitations. In addition, consideration for adopt-
> ing newer approaches, such as following ontological and precision-
> based medicine principles, accounting for genetics/epigenetic and neuro-
> biological factors, and the inclusion of biomarkers will potentially result in
> more thorough and comprehensive classification systems and diagnostic
> criteria.

Temporomandibular Joint Imaging   227

Steven R. Singer and Mel Mupparapu

> Prescriptions for imaging studies for temporomandibular disorders are
> based on the patient's complaint, history, and clinical findings. Appro-
> priate selection criteria and justification for imaging examinations must
> be followed. Because the temporomandibular joint is composed of both
> hard and soft tissues, different studies are prescribed based on the clini-
> cally suspected condition. Current imaging modalities include panoramic
> radiographs, cone-beam computed tomography, and MRI. The entire ex-
> amination must be interpreted, and the findings recorded in the patient

record. No one imaging modalities is suitable for all patients. An oral and maxillofacial radiologist should be consulted when the interpretation of the study is beyond the scope of the practitioner.

role of occlusion and occlusal disharmony in TMD etiopathogenesis. Recognition of this evidence-based literature is paramount in eliminating and preventing the chances of overtreatment of patients with TMD.

Over the past several decades, the science of restorative/reconstructive dentistry and orthodontics has evolved tremendously, following sound principles passed down from robust literature and scientific rationale. These principles have been solid and instrumental in enhancing dentistry, from a single tooth restoration to complex full-mouth rehabilitations. However, it must be noted that some of the principles and philosophies followed over these decades have been questioned based on the advances in science, technology, and evidence-based medicine. The scenario became complex when clinicians were faced with the question of guidance for optimum joint and muscle health as related to restorative dentistry and orthodontics.

This paper provided an overview of the knowledge on the relationship between temporomandibular disorders (TMDs) and the main sleep conditions and disorders of dental interest, namely, sleep bruxism (SB), sleep apnea, and gastroesophageal reflux disease (GERD). It emerged that although the topic of SB as a possible detrimental factor for the stomatognathic structures has been the most studied, evidence is growing that SB, obstructive sleep apnea, and GERD, all belong to a circle of mutually interacting sleep disorders and conditions that, in turn, may be associated with TMDs. The pathophysiology of the cause-and-effect relationships, if existing, has to be elucidated yet.

Unvalidated theories have been proposed for the etiopathogenesis of masticatory myofascial temporomandibular disorders (mTMD). Modalities such as cone-beam computed tomography/computed tomography and MRI contributes little to the diagnosis of mTMD. Diagnosing mTMD is based on the recognition of "familiar pain" presentation in the masticatory myofascial tissue. This assessment tool contributes little our understanding of the underlying disease process. Thus, management of mTMD is empirical and arbitrary. Exploring emerging technologies to identify biomarkers and objectively assess myofascial tissue physiology in disease and health may be key in moving the diagnosis of mTMD from the pragmatic paradigm to an evidence-based paradigm.

DENTAL CLINICS OF NORTH AMERICA

SERIES OF RELATED INTEREST

Atlas of the Oral and Maxillofacial Surgery Clinics
https://www.oralmaxsurgeryatlas.theclinics.com/

Oral and Maxillofacial Surgery Clinics
https://www.oralmaxsurgery.theclinics.com/

THE CLINICS ARE AVAILABLE ONLINE!
Access your subscription at:
www.theclinics.com

Erratum

In the July 2022 *Dental Clinics* (Volume 66, number 3) article, "Smile Management: A Discussion with the Masters," pages 489-501, an author's name was mistakenly transposed. The author should be listed as "Dimitris N. Tatakis, DDS, PhD."

Dent Clin N Am 67 (2023) xiii
https://doi.org/10.1016/j.cden.2023.02.002

dental.theclinics.com

Tribute

In a student's life, there are some good teachers, and then there are mentors. Dr Henry A. Gremillion was an exceptional mentor. When *Dental Clinics of North America* asked us to serve as guest editors of a special *Dental Clinics of North America* issue on temporomandibular disorders (TMDs), we thought of making it exceptionally special by dedicating this entire issue as a humble tribute to one of the finest mentors we have ever come across in dentistry. My first interaction with Henry was sometime in 2005, when I was a student in his TMJ Orofacial Pain course at the University of Florida in Gainesville. Apart from being a superb humanitarian, an outstanding clinician, and an exceptional teacher, Henry was a font of kindness and goodness.

I still vividly remember one of the days of the four-week course when I did not have a patient for my clinical portion of the course. He asked me, "Dave, you really need to get your hands wet in the clinical component. What are you going to do?" I told him it is not practical for me to fly a patient from New Jersey. What happened next was unbelievable. Henry jumped into the chair and told me to make the surface markings on his face so that I could fully experience the course. I first thought he was joking, and the jovial gesture that I made turned into total disbelief when I began to realize that he was serious. The commitment to his course, mentees, students, patients, and humanity was unique to Henry. He became my first mentor in Orofacial pain, and a dear friend. At every scientific meeting, I would wait to meet him, see that wide smile, and laugh at his practical jokes and comments. Henry, we miss you dearly in this field! Thank you for inspiring hundreds of us to excel in life in general, and in orofacial pain in particular. I am proud to have been your mentee.

Loving friends,
Steve and Dave

Davis C. Thomas, BDS, DDS, MSD, MSc Med, MSc
Department of Diagnostic Sciences
Rutgers School of Dental Medicine
110 Bergen Street, Room D885A
Newark, NJ 07103-2400, USA

Steven R. Singer, DDS
Department of Diagnostic Sciences
Rutgers School of Dental Medicine
110 Bergen Street, Room D885A
Newark, NJ 07103-2400, USA

E-mail addresses:
davisct1@gmail.com (D.C. Thomas)
singerst@sdm.rutgers.edu (S.R. Singer)

https://doi.org/10.1016/j.cden.2023.02.001
0011-8532/23/© 2023 Published by Elsevier Inc.

dental.theclinics.com

Preface

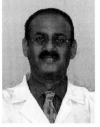
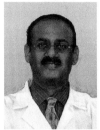

Davis C. Thomas, BDS, DDS, MSD, MSc Med, MSc   Steven R. Singer, DDS
Editors

Temporomandibular joint disorders (TMDs) encompass a broad spectrum of clinical entities that manifest with pain and/or dysfunction of the temporomandibular joints and associated structures. Since the last issue on this topic that was presented as a special issue in *Dental Clinics of North America* (January 2007), there have been substantial advances and updates in the diagnosis, classification, and management of these conditions. The robust nature of the scientific TMD literature in the last two decades demonstrates a consistent and deepening interest in this field by dental clinicians. The perfect blend of clinical dentistry and evidence-based medicine is evolving in the field of TMD, thereby enhancing patient care and improving outcome. The recognition of orofacial pain as the twelfth dental specialty by the American Dental Association makes this special issue of *Dental Clinics of North America* timely and it is hoped thought-provoking.

It is estimated that an average of 25% of Americans (80 to 90 million Americans) suffers from chronic pain. TMDs are considered the second most prevalent painful chronic musculoskeletal condition (second to low back pain) and affect between 6% and 12% of the general population. The role of the dental clinician in general, and an orofacial pain specialist, has become ever more significant, considering the pain, suffering, and the morbidity with which TMDs present. The significant association of TMDs with systemic conditions, genetics, sleep, and psychological factors has made this entity more challenging to the clinician than ever before. Concomitantly, the impressive rise in quality evidence-based studies is beginning to have its effect on significantly improved diagnosis and management of TMDs and associated comorbidities.

This special issue of *Dental Clinics of North America* brings together the world's leading experts in this field. We are honored and privileged to be editors of this issue. The interactions with stalwarts in the field of clinical TMD practice, research, and academics that has occurred during the past several months toward the preparation of this issue have been nothing short of extraordinary. It has been our distinct pleasure to have worked with such a highly scholastic group of contributors, and it is gratifying to see the quality of articles that are included. We do acknowledge that the science of

Dent Clin N Am 67 (2023) xvii–xviii
https://doi.org/10.1016/j.cden.2023.01.001
0011-8532/23/© 2023 Published by Elsevier Inc.

TMDs is a vast field, and this issue is by no means a substitute for an all-encompassing textbook on the subject. However, it is our sincere hope that this issue is thought-provoking and concomitantly sheds light on potential uncertainties and controversies in the field. We present this special issue as memoriam to Dr Henry A Gremillion, who was an outstanding TMD researcher, clinician, and mentor to hundreds of students, and a dear friend of ours.

We wish to acknowledge and thank our mentors, colleagues, residents, students, and the current contributors, without whose constant support this type of endeavor would not have been possible. We also thank our friends and families for the support during the time we had to take away from them. Our immense gratitude to John Vassallo, Ann Gielou Posedio, and the entire *Dental Clinics of North America* team for their continued and constant support.

Davis C. Thomas, BDS, DDS, MSD, MSc Med, MSc
Department of Diagnostic Sciences
Rutgers School of Dental Medicine
Newark, NJ 07103-2400, USA

Steven R. Singer, DDS
Department of Diagnostic Sciences
Rutgers School of Dental Medicine
110 Bergen Street, Room D885A
Newark, NJ 07103-2400, USA

E-mail addresses:
davisct1@gmail.com (D.C. Thomas)
singerst@sdm.rutgers.edu (S.R. Singer)

Temporomandibular Joint
Review of Anatomy and Clinical Implications

Veronica Iturriaga, DDS, MSc, PhD[a],*, Thomas Bornhardt, DDS, MSc[a],
Nicol Velasquez, DDS[b]

KEYWORDS

- Temporomandibular joint • Temporomandibular joint disorders • Mandibular condyle
- Temporomandibular joint disk • Synovial membrane • Masticatory muscles
- Anatomy

KEY POINTS

- Temporomandibular joint (TMJ) is one of the most complex joints of the human being; it allows the movement of the jaw and with it, the functions of the stomatognathic system.
- TMJ is composed of the mandibular fossa, joint tubercle, and the condylar process of the mandible, separated by an articular disk.
- TMJ is a synovial joint and is covered by the synovial membrane, responsible for secreting synovial fluid, which is responsible for joint nutrition, lubrication, and health.
- Both TMJs always work symmetrically supported by four pairs of muscles that create their movements, known as muscles of mastication.

INTRODUCTION

The masticatory or stomatognathic system has to be understood as a physiologic, functional, and perfectly defined entity composed of a heterogenous set of organs and tissue, of which biology and physiopathology are absolutely interdependent.[1] Its first sketches belong to chordate amphibians from around 550 million years ago.[2] Later, due to natural selection, the human masticatory system evolved following a common plan with vertebrate gnathostomes, where we can find two distinct units, one represented by the cranium and maxilla, and the other being the mandible.[2] Both units were derived from the first pharyngeal arch and were composed of an external osteoderm coating and a cartilaginous internal core.

[a] Department of Integral Adult Care Dentistry, Universidad de La Frontera. Francisco Salazar Avenue 01145, Temuco, Chile; [b] Temporomandibular Disorder, Orofacial Pain Program, Universidad de La Frontera. Francisco Salazar Avenue 01145, Temuco, Chile
* Corresponding author. Department of Integral Adult Care Dentistry, Universidad de La Frontera. Francisco Salazar Avenue 01145, Temuco, Chile.
E-mail address: veronica.iturriaga@ufrontera.cl

Dent Clin N Am 67 (2023) 199–209
https://doi.org/10.1016/j.cden.2022.11.003

In the evolution of the osseous components of the current temporomandibular joint (TMJ), in the first instance, the primitive square-articular or Meckelian joint was found, which evolved to become the joint of the incus and the malleus, hence its close anatomic relationship with the current TMJ. This was followed by the first form of TMJ called the squamosal dentary joint. This first form of TMJ was composed of two bones: one called temporal squama, which presented membranous ossification; and another called dentary bone, which presented endochondral ossification.[2,3] Subsequently, a change is generated at the craniofacial level, where three important events occur: (1) the adoption of an upright posture and bipedalism; (2) increased brain volume; and (3) modification of the masticatory apparatus. The latter, mainly conceived by changes in the function of the masticatory system, will generate an increase in the height of the face and muscular development that will allow the richness of movements that the system presents and gives way to one of the most complex joints of the organism.[4] For his part, Baune[1] postulated that the development of TMJs has a single embryologic origin from two blastemas, separated in space and time: the condylar blastema and the temporal or glenoid blastema. Unlike the other joints in the body, the TMJ does not have the development of its two components at the same time. Initially, in the seventh week of intrauterine life, the condylar component differentiates, while in the ninth week of intrauterine life, the temporal component differentiates; the final process culminates at the twenty-first week of gestation. Although the TMJ's two components begin their differentiation at different times, they develop in directions that approximate them. The condylar component does it posteriorly, superiorly, and laterally; while the temporal component, toward the bottom, anterior and medial.[1,3]

At the bone level, the TMJ is currently composed of the mandibular fossa (MF) and the articular tubercle (AT), both belonging to the squamous portion of the temporal bone; and the condylar process (CP) of the mandible, which includes the mandibular condyle (MC)[5,6] (**Figs. 1** and **2**). Both bones are separated by an articular disk (AD),

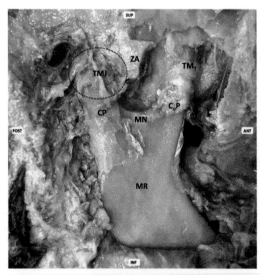

Fig. 1. Localization of the temporomandibular joint (human cadaveric specimen, sagittal view). TMJ, temporomandibular joint; C_0P, coronoid process; CP, condylar process; MN, mandibular notch; MR, mandibular ramus; TM_T, temporalis muscle tendon; ZA, zygomatic arch; Dotted circle, ANT, anterior; INF, inferior; POST, posterior; SUP, superior; TMJ localization.

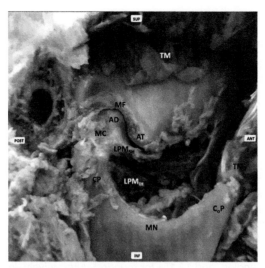

Fig. 2. Temporomandibular joint anatomy components (human cadaveric specimen, sagittal view). MF, mandibular fossa; AD, articular disk; ANT, anterior; AT, articular tubercle; C_oP, coronoid process; CP, condylar process; INF, inferior; LPM_{IH}, lateral pterygoid muscle, inferior head; LPM_{SH}, lateral pterygoid muscle, superior head; MC, mandibular condyle; MN, mandibular notch; POST, posterior; SUP, superior; TM, temporalis muscle; TM_T, temporalis muscle tendon.

which is formed by fibrous connective tissue with islands of fibrocartilage devoid of blood vessels or nerve fibers in its center.[5] Various ligaments and muscle tissue are attached to this structure, which will provide stability and movement, respectively.

According to the above, the objective of this article was to review the anatomy of the TMJ and its adjoining structures from a clinical perspective. First, we review the general characteristics of the TMJ, then its bony, cartilaginous, ligamentous, and synovial components, and finally the muscles that are related to the TMJ.

GENERAL CHARACTERISTICS OF THE TEMPOROMANDIBULAR JOINT

On a sagittal plane, the TMJ is anatomically located in the middle region of the head, being a union point for the temporal, cranial, and mandibular regions. This joint allows the movement of the mandible and consequently gives way to all the functions of the stomatognathic system. On a coronal plane, we can find two TMJs, one on the far right of the face and one on the far left, sharing the mandibular bone. Because of this, both TMJs function as a complex, where the movement of one joint will affect the contralateral TMJ. The TMJ presents a mean depth from the skin to the lateral pole of the MC of approximately 17 mm, with a high correlation between the depth of the right and left sides. However, no correlation has been found between TMJ depth and age or sex.[7] It is important to mention that the complex formed by both TMJ will confront the maxillary bone with the mandibular bone and, therefore, will be related to the occlusion of the teeth, being linked to the growth and development of these structures throughout life.

The TMJ is classified as a synovial joint, which is characterized by presenting a space called the articular cavity, which is delimited by an articular capsule (AC). The AC has a thin membrane that covers its internal portion, which is called synovium or synovial membrane (SM) and is responsible for secreting synovial fluid (SF). The SF is responsible for the nutrition, lubrication, and health of the joint.[5,8]

OSSEOUS AND CARTILAGINOUS COMPONENTS OF THE TEMPOROMANDIBULAR JOINT
Condylar Process and Mandibular Condyle

The TMJ comprises the CP of the mandibular bone and the AT and MF belonging to the temporal bone. The CP of the mandibular bone belongs to the mandibular ramus and is a prolongation that extends rostrally from the mandibular notch, passing through the condylar neck and ending in the MC (see **Figs. 1** and **2**). The latter represents the portion that belongs to the TMJ and is defined as an eminence whose major axis is oriented obliquely posteriorly and medially, approximately 20° to the coronal plane[6]; it has a longer ellipsoidal convex shape lateromedially than anteroposteriorly, approximately 15 to 20 mm and 8 to 10 mm, respectively.[6,9] In a sagittal view, the MC has a posterior and medial direction, and its functional surfaces are represented by its superior and anterior zone. These features are responsible for the TMJ being classified as a condylar or ellipsoidal joint.[5]

Four physiologic condylar shapes have been described which are flat, convex, angled, and round. According to Yale and colleagues,[6] 97.1% of all condyles fall into one of these four groups, with relative frequencies of 27.2% for flat, 43.3% for convex, 13.4% for angled, and 12.1% for rounded. Alternatively, in a study by Oberg and colleagues,[10] where 102 TMJs of skulls between 20 and 93 years of age were analyzed, it was observed that from a frontal plane, the most predominant shape was rounded or slightly convex (55%), followed by the flat shape (20%) and an inverted "V" shape or other shapes (25%). In clinical practice, we can also find some alterations in the shape and condylar development, with the bifid shape or bifid condyle being one of the most frequent anatomic variations. Two possible causes for the bifid condyle are described; the first one was described by Blackwood (1957), where it is postulated that the presence of a bifid condyle is associated with the embryologic maintenance or preservation of a fibrovascular loop or septum in the MC, which divides the growth of this in two; usually, these septa are present in the condylar cartilage until week 20 of the embryonic development. The other theory was presented by Thomason and Yusuf, which describes the appearance of the bifid condyle occurring at a later stage of development associated with trauma and consequent condylar fracture, which would cause a medial or lateral displacement of the MC, generating growth and adaptation of the fracture trait, transforming into a pseudo-condyle.[11-13] Other alterations that can affect the CP, the temporal bone components, and the AD are the agenesis, hypoplasia, and hyperplasia of these tissues.

The MC has a lateral pole and a medial pole. The lateral pole is rough, with a blunt tip,[9] and is linked to the lateral collateral ligament and the lateral ligament (LL) (formerly called temporomandibular ligament). Instead, the medial pole is smooth and round and is where the medial collateral ligament is inserted. Also, the condylar neck is part of the insertion of important ligamentous and muscular structures, and the AC is inserted around it. On its anteromedial side is the pterygoid fovea, an anatomic region of clinical importance since a large part of the upper portion of the lateral pterygoid muscle and all of its lower portions are inserted[6] (see **Fig. 2**). Similarly, in the lateral area of the CP, fibers of the masseter muscle are inserted in its deep superior portion, and in the medial area of the CP, fibers of the medial pterygoid muscle are inserted. Therefore, from a clinical practice point of view, the TMJ is a meeting point between the different muscles involved in mastication, which, based on trigeminal motor control, will give way to complex mandibular movements.

Mandibular Fossa and Articular Tubercule

In the cranial structure, the components of the TMJ correspond to the MF and the AT. The MF is located in the squamous portion of the temporal bone. It is a concave structure that, when extended anteriorly, forms a convex structure, which corresponds to the AT that belongs to the zygomatic process of the temporal bone[6] (see **Fig. 2**). In this way, the anterior slope of the MF corresponds to the same anatomic place as the posterior slope of the AT. The MF presents a posterior and medial direction from a sagittal cut, as does the MC. In the posterosuperior area, it is traversed by the petrotympanic fissure and the tympanosquamous fissure, which delimit the functional portion of the MF anteriorly. The functional portion of the AT extends up to 5 mm anterior to its apex. Therefore, it is in these functional zones where the CM moves in the different mandibular movements. The MF has no bony wall laterally, but this area is reinforced by the AC and the LL. Unlike the lateral zone, the medial zone of the MF does present a bony wall, which is related to the medial pole of the MC.

The functional surfaces of the MC, MF, and AT are covered by fibrocartilage, unlike the other synovial joints, which are covered by hyaline cartilage. These functional surfaces have thicknesses of approximately 1.5 to 2 mm in the MC and 0.5 to 1 mm in the MF and AT[9,14] (**Fig. 3**). Fibrocartilage is a tissue rich in collagen fibers associated with cartilaginous tissue and gives the TMJ a greater capacity to withstand friction during joint movements and a better repair capacity against adaptive conditions. Fibrocartilage presents three distinct histologic zones. The first one, often called the superficial, tangential, or articular area, is the outermost layer and is covered by dense fibrous connective tissue with type I and type III collagen, with little fibroblast-like cellularity. In this layer, the fibers are parallel to the surface and are tightly bound to withstand the forces of movement. The second layer, called the middle, transitional, proliferative or cellular zone, is composed of undifferentiated cells and spherical chondrocytes in a matrix of proteoglycans, which gives the articular cartilage the possibility of proliferation, allowing the TMJ to respond to functional demands and loads. The third layer, called the deep, radial, or cartilaginous zone, is the thickest of the three layers. It mainly presents lacunae of chondrocytes organized in isogenic groups with some intertwined type I and III collagen fibers and other fibers in a radial manner; it also presents hypertrophic chondrocytes, although deeper. For its part, below the fibrocartilage described above is calcified cartilage, which presents necrotic hypertrophic chondrocytes surrounded by a calcified matrix, which gives way to the subchondral bone with predominating blood elements in its bone marrow. **Fig. 3** shows the different histologic layers and some of their main components.

Articular Disk

The AD is a fibrocartilage structure that lies between the surfaces of the MC, MF, and AT. From a histologic point of view, the disk is a structure of avascular fibrous cartilage with a predominance of type I collagen fibers arranged in parallel and chondrocytes stacked in columns that follow the direction of the collagen fibers. These rows of chondrocytes become more abundant and denser toward the peripheral zone of the AD (see **Fig. 3**). It has a concave-convex shape toward the upper and lower part, with a thinner central zone, which thickens toward the periphery (see **Fig. 2**). Its thicknesses are 3 mm in the posterior sector, 2 mm in the anterior, and 1 mm in the intermediate area.[9,14] From a sagittal view, the AD has a thick posterior zone that, at rest, will be linked to the highest part of the MF and the top of the MC. It also presents a middle zone, which, as mentioned, is the thinnest and, at rest, is linked to the anterior slope of the MF and the anterosuperior zone of the MC. The anterior part is of intermediate thickness and is linked, in a state of rest, to the anterior slope of the MF, the AT, and

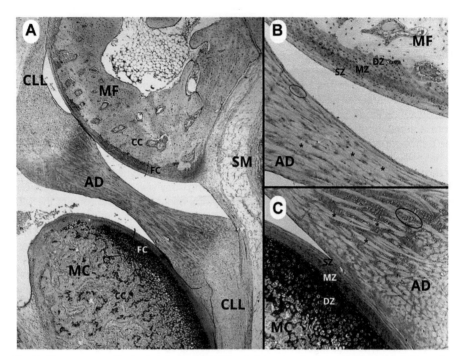

Fig. 3. Temporomandibular joint of rabbit (*Oryctolagus cuniculus*). (*A*). Sagittal section of a general view of the joint, magnification 2.5x. (*B*). Sagittal section focused on the supradiscal compartment, articular disk and mandibular fossa, 10x magnification. (*C*). Sagittal section focused on the infradiscal compartment, articular disk and mandibular condyle, 10x magnification. AD, articular disk; CC, calcified cartilage; DZ, deep zone; MC, mandibular condyle; MF, Mandibular fossa; MZ, mid-zone; SM, synovial membrane; SZ, superficial zone; Oval circle, chondrocytes arranged in clusters parallel to the collagen fibers; Asterisk, collagen fibers in parallel with each other. Toluidine Blue stain.

the anterior area of the MC. When performing opening, lateral or protrusion movements, the disk will change its location to place its thinner avascular and aneural medial zone between the functional surfaces of the MF, AT and MC, accompanying the condyle in its movements. It is important to mention that a large part of the superior lateral pterygoid muscle head, as well as fibers of the inferior lateral pterygoid muscle head, are inserted in the anterior area of the AD. From a clinical perspective, there are some controversies regarding these insertions, suggesting that some disk displacements could be related to this disk-muscular union. However, it has been determined that the position of the AD depends mainly on its shape, inter-articular pressure, and lubrication, so this relationship is still under study.

Regarding collateral ligaments, these attach the lateral and medial pole to the AD, acting as an intermediate bridge, explaining why this structure is called disk and not meniscus, allowing some movement of the AD during mandibular dynamics. This situation leads to two virtual spaces, a larger superior or supradiscal joint space, and a smaller inferior or infradiscal joint space. The superior joint space is traditionally related to the translation movements of the MC on the MF, and the inferior joint space is related to condylar rotation movements.[9,14] In any case, it is crucial to consider that joint movement presents a constant roto-translation. In some disk-condylar pathologies, the articular spaces may be compromised, for example, in disk perforations or displacements, in which, as a consequence of joint inflammation, edema or effusion may occur. Currently, with some minimally invasive procedures, treating these spaces more specifically is possible, resulting in a more personalized therapeutic management of the condition.

LIGAMENTS AND SYNOVIAL MEMBRANE OF THE TEMPOROMANDIBULAR JOINT

The TMJ is surrounded by a connective tissue called AC, which is more fibrous laterally and looser medially. The AC is cone shaped. It originates from the zygomatic process of the temporal bone, from the tympanosquamosal fissure to in front of the AT in a superficial plane, and from the base of the spine of the sphenoid bone in a deep plane. It extends inferiorly and posteriorly, covering the whole TMJ and inserting into the neck of the MC.[4,8,15] The AC acts by resisting forces that try to separate or dislocate the joint surfaces. It is important to mention that the AC is directly related to the collateral ligaments; it is even said that these would be an extension of this tissue. It is also related to the AD, LL, and all muscle attachments found in the area. The inner area of the AC is lined by a loose connective tissue membrane called SM, which confines and produces the SF. This membrane has villi and extensions toward the articular cavity, associating with the supradiscal and infradiscal spaces to deliver nutrition, lubrication, and health to the joint tissues. These folds increase in number with age, as well as in pathologic processes, mainly inflammatory ones. The SM has two layers, the subintimal, fibrovascular or subsynovial layer, which is attached to the fibrous connective tissue of the AC and has a network of capillaries with some lymphatic vessels; and the intimate synovial layer that is related to the articular space, presenting both phagocytic or type A synoviocytes, and secretory or type B synoviocytes. Secretory synoviocytes are responsible for producing SF, which is a yellowish viscous gel, similar to egg white, that has regulatory, metabolic, and lubricating functions. The TMJ has two forms of lubrication: limit lubrication which occurs during mandibular movements, driving the SF from the margins or synovial recesses to the articular surface; and exudative lubrication, which occurs in joint compression and decompression movements, making the SF soak the surfaces like a sponge, favoring metabolic exchange. The SF has a virtual volume of 1 mL and contains various plasma proteins, lipids, sugars, cellular components, cytokines, growth factors, proteolytic enzymes, lubricating molecules, and others. Of these components, the lubricating molecules stand out, among which hyaluronic acid and lubricin are the main ones.[16] Using these elements is how some currently used therapies seek to restore joint health in inflammatory processes or osteoarthritis by supplementing exogenous hyaluronic acid, promoting visco-induction, viscosupplementation and immunomodulation.

Similarly, if we continue with the ligamentous components, we find the LL, whose function is to reinforce the lateral area of the TMJ. The LL is a fibrous connective tissue structure that is traditionally divided into two portions: (1) a deep, short, horizontal portion running from the AT to the lateral pole of the MC; and (2) a more extensive and superficial oblique portion, which goes from the zygomatic arch downwards and posteriorly to be inserted in the posterior part of the condylar neck and mandibular ramus. Some authors also describe a medial or internal temporomandibular ligament, which would extend obliquely from the spine of the sphenoid to the neck of the MC; however, its description is scarce.[15] Another intrinsic ligament of great importance is the posterior ligament or bilaminar zone, previously called retrodiscal tissue. This structure has elastic fibers in its upper part that join the AD with the posterior part of the MF, and collagen fibers in its lower part that join the disk to the condylar neck. Both fibers form something similar to a cushion, which is related to the posterior part of the AC, which would be an entry point for vascular and neural tissues.

MAIN MUSCLE COMPONENTS RELATED TO THE TEMPOROMANDIBULAR JOINT

Like any other type of joint, the TMJ itself cannot make movements; therefore, for the TMJ to move, it needs the action of associated muscles. These muscles are called masticatory muscles, one of the main muscle groups of the head. Masticatory muscles are four pairs that work in a coordinated manner to produce mandibular movement[17] and correspond to the masseter, temporalis, medial pterygoid, and lateral pterygoid muscles.

Embryologically, masticatory muscles develop from the first pharyngeal arch or mandibular arch, together with the mandibular cartilage (or Meckel's) and the trigeminal nerve. Therefore, masticatory muscles are motor innervated by one of the branches of the trigeminal nerve, specifically the anterior trunk of the mandibular nerve. Furthermore, they are mainly supplied by branches of the maxillary artery. They are all paired muscles located on each side of the head, and from their origin, they extend to be inserted into the rami of the mandible to produce all mandibular movements in conjunction with the TMJ complex.[9,17]

The primary masticatory muscle is the masseter, and it is the most superficial and palpable. It is rectangular and elongated from superior to inferior, occupying the thickness of an anatomic region known as the masseteric region. Two portions form it; a superficial fascicle, whose fibers have a descending and slightly oblique course toward the back, and a deep fascicle, formed by vertical fibers (**Fig. 4**). Some authors describe the presence of three fascicles: one superficial, another deep, and another intermediate.[17] It originates from the lower border and the anterior two-thirds of the zygomatic arch. Its

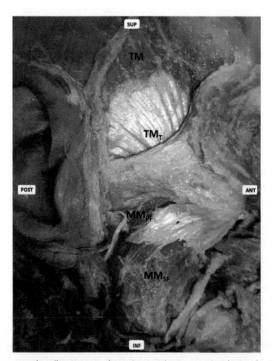

Fig. 4. Masticatory muscles (human cadaveric specimen, sagittal view). ANT, anterior; INF, inferior; MM$_{PF}$, masseter fasciculus profundus muscle; MM$_{SF}$, masseter fasciculus superficialis muscle; POST, posterior; SUP, superior; TM, temporalis muscle; TM$_{T}$, temporalis muscle tendon.

fibers converge inferiorly to insert on the outer face of the ramus of the mandible and the mandibular angle. When this muscle contracts, it causes a robust elevation of the jaw, and the teeth come into contact; In addition, the superficial fascicle, due to the direction of its fibers, is related to the mandibular protrusive movements.[9,17,18]

Similarly, the temporalis muscle is a flat, radiated, fan-shaped muscle with anterior fibers that are vertically oriented, middle fibers that are obliquely oriented, and posterior fibers that are somewhat horizontally oriented. Its origin is in the temporal fossa of the skull and the deep surface of the temporal fascia, at the level of the inferior temporal line. The muscle fibers converge inferiorly, forming a tendon that emerges from the temporal fossa, passes inferior to the zygomatic arch, and inserts into the coronoid process, anterior border of the mandibular ramus, as well as the medial and lateral borders of the retromolar fossa.[17,19] (see **Fig. 4**). The anterior and middle fibers of the temporalis muscle are used to elevate the mandible, and the posterior fibers produce mandibular retrusion. In mandibular closure, this muscle is considered an important stabilizer of movement.

The medial pterygoid muscle is a thick, rectangular muscle parallel to the masseter muscle, but positioned on the inner face of the mandible. It originates at the pterygoid fossa level located in the sphenoid bone's pterygoid processes. Its muscular body is oblique downwards, posteriorly, and laterally, inserting into the inner side of the mandibular angle and ramus.[17] This muscle and the masseter muscle form a muscular sling around the inferior border and angle of the mandible, thus working together for mandibular elevation and protrusion. This muscle also participates in lateral movements, where unilateral contraction will produce a mandibular mediotrusion movement.

Lastly, the lateral pterygoid muscle is the primary muscle of the infratemporal fossa. It comprises two portions: an upper head and a lower head. On the one hand, the superior head is considerably smaller than the inferior head, originating from the infratemporal surface of the greater wing of the sphenoid bone; it extends almost horizontally, posteriorly, and laterally until its insertion in the AC, AD, and condylar neck.[17] Regarding the percentage of fibers that are inserted into the AD, it has been established mainly by histologic techniques and magnetic resonance imaging that the percentages of insertion vary from 29.5% to 69.3%.[20] On the other hand, the inferior head of lateral pterygoid muscle originates on the outer face of the external wing of the pterygoid process and extends posteriorly, superiorly, and laterally to insert into the pterygoid fovea on the condylar neck. When the inferior bundles contract bilaterally, the MCs are tractioned by them, sliding anteriorly and inferiorly across the ATs, producing protrusion of the mandible. If to this movement is added the effect of the mandibular depressor muscles, mandibular descent or opening will be generated. Unilateral contraction creates lateral movement of the mandible to the opposite side. When the lower bundle acts during the opening, the upper head remains inactive, only coming into action in conjunction with the levator muscles.

As described, the TMJs always work symmetrically, supported by these four pairs of muscles that create their movements. When the TMJs work properly, the different movements can be performed without pain or discomfort. However, the mandibular movements can be affected when the TMJ presents some pathology. In the same way, the muscles can perceive some joint alteration, producing a protective co-contraction and even the maintenance of this and subsequent muscular pathology.

SUMMARY

The TMJ is one of the most important and complex joints in the human being. Each is located at one end of the face: however, both work as morpho-functional sets. In this way, the anatomy of the TMJ and its associated structures will influence the mandible's dynamics and function, so an alteration of its components can cause deterioration of the system and subsequent disease. Knowledge of the normal anatomy is fundamental for the clinical approach, allowing differentiation between the healthy and the sick.

CLINICS CARE POINTS

TMJ is anatomically located in the middle region of the head in sagittal view, being a union point for the temporal, cranial, and mandibular regions. Is composed of the MF, AT, and CP of the mandible, separated by an articular disk. TMJ allows the movement of the mandible and consequently gives way to all the functions of the stomatognathic system.

Articular disk has a thick posterior zone that, at rest, is linked to the highest part of the MF and the top of the MC. Also presents a middle zone, which is the thinnest and, at rest, is linked to the anterior slope of the MF and the anterosuperior zone of the MC. During movements, the disk will change its location to place its thinner avascular and aneural medial zone between the functional surfaces of the MF, AT, and MC, accompanying the condyle in its movements.

The TMJ is classified as a synovial joint, composed of an AC and an SM that is responsible for secreting SF. SF is synthesized by synoviocytes and is composed of various molecules among which lubricating molecules such as hyaluronic acid and lubricin stand out. Thus, SF is responsible for the nutrition, lubrication, and health of the joint.

TMJs always work symmetrically, supported by these four pairs of muscles that create their movements. Because of this, both TMJs function as a complex, where the movement of one joint will affect the contralateral TMJ. When the TMJs work properly, the different movements can be performed without pain or discomfort, but the mandibular movements can be affected when the TMJ presents some pathology.

DISCLOSURE

All authors contributed to the conception and design of the study, drafting the article, critically revising the manuscript for important intellectual content, and giving final approval and agreeing to be accountable for all aspects of this work.

Role of the funding source: The study was financed by Project DI20-0018 and the Temporomandibular Disorder and Orofacial Pain Program, Universidad de La Frontera, Chile.

Conflict of interest: The authors declare that they have no conflict of interest.

REFERENCES

1. Mejia C, Salazar L. Desarrollo ontogénico de la articulación temporomandibular durante el período fetal. Rev Estomat 1996;72:15–26.
2. Gonzáles H. Origen y evolución del sistema estomatognático. In: Manns A, editor. Sistema Estomatognático. Bases biológicas y correlaciones clínicas. 1th Edition. Madrid: Ripano S.A.; 2011. p. 55–67.
3. Quijano Y. Anatomía clínica de la articulación temporomandibular. Morfolia 2011; 3:23–33.
4. Okeson J. Management of temporomandibular disorders and occlusion. 7th Edition. Barcelona: Elsevier; 2013. p. 7–14.
5. Vasconcellos H, Sousa E, Cavalcante M. Temporomandibular joint classification: functional and anatomic aspects. Int J Odontostomat 2007;1:25–8.

6. Fuentes R, Cantín M, Ottone N, et al. Characterization of bone components of the temporomandibular joint. a literature review. Int J Morphol 2015;33:1569–76.

7. Iturriaga V, Bornhardt T, Wen S, et al. Mandibular condyle depth analysis in magnetic resonance of patients with temporomandibular disorders. Int J Morphol 2020;38:458–60.

8. Gomez de Ferraris M. Histología y embriología bucodental. 2nd Edition. Santiago de Chile: Panamericana; 2009. p. 190–9.

9. Alomar X, Medrano J, Cabratosa J, et al. Anatomy of the temporomandibular joint. Semin Ultrasound CT MR 2007;28:170–83.

10. Bumann A, Lotzmann U. TMJ disorders and orofacial pain the role of dentistry in a multidisciplinary diagnostic approach. Color atlas of dental medicine. Stuttgart, Germany: Thieme; 2002. p. 18–9.

11. Blackwood H. The double headed mandibular condyle. Amer J Phys Antropol 1957;15:1–8.

12. Thomason J, Yusuf H. Traumatically induced bifid mandibular condyle: a report of two cases. Br Dent J 1986;25:291–3.

13. De Sales M, do Amaral J, de Amorim R, et al. Bifid Mandibular condyle: case report and etiological considerations. J Can Dent Assoc 2004;70:158–62.

14. Castellano J, Navano R, Santana R, et al. Fisiología de la articulación temporomandibular. Canar méd quir 2006;4:10–6.

15. Fuentes R, Ottone N, Bucchi C, et al. Analysis of terms used in the literature to refer to temporomandibular joint capsule and joint ligaments. Int J Morphol 2016;34:342–50.

16. Iturriaga V, Mena P, Oliveros R, et al. Value of synovial fluid in the temporomandibular joint and its implications in articular pathology. Int J Morphol 2018;36:297–302.

17. Basit H, Tariq M, Siccardi M. Anatomy, head and neck: mastication muscles. In: Statpearls publishing. 2022. Available at: https://www.statpearls.com/ArticleLibrary/viewarticle/24766. Accessed July 24, 2022.

18. Corcoran N, Goldman E. Anatomy, head and neck: masseter muscle. In: Statpearls publishing. 2022. Available at: https://www.statpearls.com/ArticleLibrary/viewarticle/36340. Accessed July 24, 2022.

19. Bressler H, Markus M, Bressler R, et al. Temporal tendinosis: a cause of chronic orofacial pain. Curr Pain Headache Rep 2020;24:1–9.

20. Farfán C, Roig J, Quidel B, et al. Morphological and functional analysis of the lateral pterygoid muscle: a review of the literature. Int J Morphol 2020;38:1713–21.

Classification and Diagnosis of Temporomandibular Disorders and Temporomandibular Disorder Pain

Gary D. Klasser, DMD[a],*, Jean-Paul Goulet, DDS, MSD, FRCD[b],
Isabel Moreno-Hay, DDS PhD ABOP ABDSM[c]

KEYWORDS

- Classification systems • Diagnostic criteria • Temporomandibular disorders (TMD)
- Orofacial pain

KEY POINTS

- Classification systems are essential because they provide a conceptual framework of information that stems from our understanding of the etiology, pathophysiology, and features of diseases and disorders specific to a field of interest to improve the quality of diagnosis and patient management.
- There is no consensus regarding a unique and universal classification of temporomandibular disorders (TMD); however, the breadth of clinical entities under the umbrella term "temporomandibular disorders" is best captured for now within the classification scheme proposed by the American Academy of Orofacial Pain.
- To date, the Diagnostic Criteria for Temporomandibular Disorders remains universally accepted as a reliable evidence-based diagnostic system for common TMD.
- The integration of ontology principles, relevant genetics/epigenetics vulnerability factors, neurobiological processes, and biomarkers represent promising steps toward the future development of a treatment-oriented classification system for TMD.

[a] Department of Diagnostic Sciences, School of Dentistry, Louisiana State University Health Sciences Center, 1100 Florida Avenue, Box #8, New Orleans, LA 70119, USA; [b] Pavillon de Médecine Dentaire, Université Laval, 2420 Rue de La Terrasse, Québec, G1V 0A6, Canada; [c] Orofacial Pain, College of Dentistry, University of Kentucky, Kentucky Clinic, Room E214, 740 S Limestone, Lexington, KY 40536, USA
* Corresponding author.
E-mail address: gklass@lsuhsc.edu

Dent Clin N Am 67 (2023) 211–225
https://doi.org/10.1016/j.cden.2022.12.001
0011-8532/23/© 2022 Elsevier Inc. All rights reserved.

dental.theclinics.com

INTRODUCTION

Currently, classification is broadly defined as a "systematic arrangement in groups or categories according to established criteria."[1] More specifically, classification systems can be viewed as a set of disease characteristics used to group individuals into a well-defined relatively homogenous population with similar clinical disease features.[2] These systems are essential for understanding disease pathogenesis and assessing treatment response. The allure of following a classification system is that it simplifies the definition of specific entities according to specific characteristics. The basis to do so is derived from an understanding and comprehension of the etiology, pathophysiology, diagnosis, and/or management of a specific disease or disorder. It must be remembered that classification systems are not intended to capture the whole universe of possible patients, but rather to capture most of the patients with key shared features of the condition. For a classification system to be ideal,[3] the following requirements would have to be met: it should be exhaustive (comprising all clinical diseases or disorders belonging to the field of interest), biologically plausible (the symptoms and signs should match with known biological processes), mutually exclusive (there should be no overlap between disease entities because of common symptoms), clinically useful (so that it can be used to help in treatment and prognosis), reliable (consistently applicable in a reproducible way between clinicians and over time) and simple for practical use.

Several organizations and individuals have developed classification systems for temporomandibular disorders (TMD), which according to the American Association for Orofacial Pain (AAOP) is defined as "A group of musculoskeletal and neuromuscular conditions that involve the TMJs, the masticatory muscles, and all associated tissues".[4] Although TMDs represent a primary cause of nonodontogenic pain in the orofacial region with pain being one of the most common and limiting clinical manifestations of such disorders, it should be realized that to be labeled with having TMD does not strictly imply this to be a painful condition. There are several conditions that may simply be viewed as annoyances rather than being painful.[5] Unfortunately, all TMD classification systems, of past and present, share the commonality of having inherent shortcomings in at least one of these qualifying requirements listed previously.

Diagnosis may be defined as the determination of the nature of an illness by evaluation of the signs, symptoms, and supportive tests in an individual patient to identify a specific disorder. Diagnostic criteria are a conglomeration of signs, symptoms, or supportive tests used in routine clinical workup to aid in a clinical diagnosis of an individual patient. Diagnostic criteria are generally broad and must reflect the different features of a disease (heterogeneity), with a view to accurately identify as many people with the condition as possible. During the care of the individual patient, diagnostic criteria may be first used to guide medical/dental care and second to help the patient gain an understanding of the disease process with prognosis. Given this complexity, the development and validation of diagnostic criteria can be quite challenging.[6,7]

Classification systems and diagnostic criteria for TMD have been developed, often based on expert opinion and the best available knowledge with their focus most often derived from particular organ systems or pathophysiological processes. Several organizations created task forces of experts to share their knowledge and experience and develop a restricted set of criteria to denominate a set of particular diagnoses organized within a hierarchical approach. Validated diagnostic criteria were used if available and if absent, criteria were formulated and supplemented with commentary explaining that data-driven criteria (validated through high-quality studies on diagnostic accuracy) are, to date, lacking. Unfortunately, this approach creates less-than-ideal situations as selected signs and symptoms and criteria are used to characterize an already selected group thus allowing for an overlapping of disease entities and contributing to heterogeneity. Moreover, if a group of patients are selected based on specific criteria, it is not known whether they all belong to a single disease or that it is a sample of (partially) overlapping disease entities. Finally, the possibility of circular reasoning exists when a criterion for selecting a group of symptomatic individuals becomes part of the diagnostic criteria defining the presence or absence of a specific disease or disorder. These issues will be further elaborated upon as individual classification systems and diagnostic criteria are discussed.

Classification systems and diagnostic criteria, although seem to be different, essentially work by complementing each other. An analogy to this process would be that of a filing system. This system includes a filing cabinet that represents the broader more encompassing classification system. The folders and files within the filing cabinet embody all diseases and disorders pertaining to a specific field according to specific criteria that distinguish each individual condition contained therein from one to another.

Classification systems and diagnostic criteria allow the clinician to follow a structured and logical approach (similar to a roadmap) thereby facilitating the accurate naming and classifying of a specific disease. This is the precursor to developing interventional approaches and strategies for patient management and thus providing a platform for discussing a prognosis with the patient. From the patient perspective, this approach results in the patient, receiving a clear and definitive diagnosis which ultimately allows for a better understanding and acceptance of aspects related to etiology and pathophysiology, promotes inclusion to a specific group, and facilitates acceptance of the various management strategies. Furthermore, it accommodates the growth of the scientific process, as researchers are able to use homogenous samples when designing clinical studies. It promotes the ability for every patient entered into a research project to be categorized according to specific and established set(s) of diagnostic criteria. Lastly, it enables all stakeholders to use a common language, thereby enhancing collaborative efforts using establishing clear terminology that will allow communication and data sharing in an unambiguous manner.

CLASSIFICATION SYSTEMS FOR TEMPOROMANDIBULAR DISORDERS
International Classification of Diseases-11th Revision by the World Health Organization

For over a century, the International Classification of Diseases (ICD) has been the reference base for gathering health statistics information and understanding the cause of death. The ICD 11th revision endorsed by the World Health Organization (WHO) in 2019 has recently come into effect.[8] The ICD is a fully electronic database that enables the assembly of large volumes of data for widespread use on the extent and consequence of human diseases. Diseases and disorders in this conceptual framework are spread across 28 top-level ICD chapters (categories) reflecting major aspects of diseases and divided into subgroups. The ICD has categories for diseases, disorders, syndromes, signs, symptoms, findings, injuries, external causes of morbidity and mortality, factors influencing health status, reasons for encounter with the health system, and traditional medicine. TMD are scattered across a large volume of anatomically, etiologically, or phenotypically defined diseases and disorders and an entity may be classified in more than one category. Entering "temporomandibular joint pain" in the coding tool leads to "Temporomandibular joint disorders" in Chapter 15, Diseases of the musculoskeletal system or connective tissue, and to "Headache or orofacial pain associated with chronic secondary temporomandibular disorders" in Chapter 21, Symptoms, signs or clinical findings, not elsewhere classified.

Among the significant improvements of the ICD 11 is the addition in Chapter 21 of a systematic classification for chronic pain of any source which is then subdivided into primary and secondary pain disorders as defined by the International Association for the Study of Pain (IASP).[9] Chronic primary TMD pain refers to pain without an established cause, although substantial knowledge may exist regarding the pathophysiological mechanisms, whereas chronic secondary TMD pain refers to pain with a known etiology and pathophysiology.[10,11] Therefore, ICD 11 allows the coding of individual TMD entities. However, as they are not all regrouped into a single chapter, it is not a classification system that enables clinicians to capture at a glance the scope of TMD conditions.

ACTTION-APS Pain Taxonomy

The limitations with existing classification systems inspired the Analgesic, Anesthetic, and Addiction Clinical Trial Translations, Innovations, Opportunities, and Networks (ACTTION) to develop a new evidence-based classification scheme for chronic pain, taking into account consequential biopsychosocial mechanisms. In partnership with the American Pain Society (APS) and the US Food and Drug Administration, this endeavor led to the 2014 publication of their collaborative taxonomy (AAPT), which is a multidimensional classification framework for chronic pain disorders.[3]

To guide clinicians toward tailored pain management and better outcomes, the AAPT categorizes chronic pain disorders into five organ systems/anatomic structures: (1) Peripheral and central nervous systems, (2) Musculoskeletal pain system, (3) Orofacial and head pain system, (4) Visceral, pelvic, and urogenital pain, (5) Disease-associated pains not classified elsewhere. Each is further divided into subcategories. For instance, "Temporomandibular disorders," "Headache disorders," and "Other orofacial pain" are specific subcategories in the "Orofacial and head pain system." The AAPT framework further characterized individual entities of chronic pain according to five dimensions: (1) core diagnostic criteria; (2) common features; (3) common medical and psychiatric comorbidities; (4) neurobiological, psychosocial, and functional consequences; and (5) putative neurobiologic and psychosocial mechanisms, risk factors, and protective factors.

Since its inception, the AAPT framework has been used for fibromyalgia and peripheral neuropathic pain conditions (ie, postherpetic neuralgia, persistent posttraumatic neuropathic pain, complex regional pain disorder, and trigeminal neuralgia).[12,13] A recent initiative led to the development of a multidimensional framework adapted for acute pain conditions (AAAPT). "Surgical/Procedural" and "Nonsurgical" are the top-level categories with fourteen and seven subcategories based on organ systems and anatomic location.[14] The five-dimensional structures retained for characterizing acute pain are (1) core criteria, (2) common features, (3) modulating factors, (4) impact/functional consequences, and (5) putative pain pathophysiologic mechanisms.

The AAPT and AAAPT offer a sound blueprint framework for building a comprehensive multiaxial classification that would complement, beyond the physical axis, the diagnosis of pain-related TMD included in the International Classification of Orofacial Pain (ICOP) and the AAOP taxonomy. Moreover, adapting the AAPT and AAAPT framework dimensions for non-painful TMD could benefit researchers and clinicians and help patient management. However, the full spectrum of TMD is still best captured and outlined in the classification system proposed by the AAOP.

American Academy of Orofacial Pain

The AAOP classification system for TMD has gained widespread dissemination and acceptance among clinicians through the AAOP Guidelines 6th edition (2018) manual.[4]

The current classification stemmed from the need for an agreed-upon TMD classification for systematic use by clinicians and researchers. The work taking place under the initiative of the International RDC/TMD Consortium of the IADR (renamed to INfORM – International Network for Orofacial Pain and Related Disorders Methodology) in partnership with the Orofacial and Head Pain Special Interest Group (OFHP SIG) of the IASP, the AAOP, the National Institute of Dental and Craniofacial Research (NIDCR), and the AAOP sister European and Australian Academies led to the consensus-based expanded TMD taxonomy published in the AAOP Guidelines manual in 2013. An overview of the methods and process of this successful endeavor has been previously presented.[15] Based on the AAOP 2008 classification scheme, TMD are sorted according to the anatomic source of signs and symptoms into joint disorders and masticatory muscle disorders. Before 2013, the AAOP classification for TMD included up to 21 individual entities compared with 52 in the current edition. The AAOP classification regroups clinical entities under joint and muscle disorders into empirically-derived categories tied to clinical features or pathophysiologic processes (**Table 1**).

To foster exchange with medical communities, the AAOP provides the corresponding *ICD* codes for each TMD (ICD 10th Revision). The AAOP classification allows going further than the original expanded TMD taxonomy when an *ICD* code exists for subtyping a disorder based on etiology. For example, there are three subtypes for orofacial dyskinesia and two for oromandibular dystonia. A retrospective look at the iterations of the AAOP TMD taxonomy exemplified the evolving nature of a classification system as new knowledge emerges. Although the AAOP classification does not include all TMD and is unrelated to etiology, it remains the best available reference. Besides capturing the scope and breadth of TMD, it also provides diagnostic criteria based on history, clinical features, and specific tests for all TMD listed, for which validity is established for the most frequent joint and muscle conditions.

American Academy of Craniofacial Pain

In 2009, the AACP published a guidelines manual for assessing, diagnosing, and managing craniofacial pain. There are three chapters devoted to conditions attributed to TMD. One chapter outlines extracapsular TMD, another deals with temporomandibular joint disorders, and the third chapter discusses myofascial pain.[16] For TMD, the AACP uses the classification published by Pertes and Gross in 1995, which separates TMD into three groups: (1) Temporomandibular joint disorders, (2) Masticatory muscle disorders, and (3) Congenital and developmental disorders.[17] The thirteen conditions under temporomandibular joint disorders are regrouped into six subcategories according to disease processes (ie, Inflammatory conditions, Degenerative diseases, Ankylosis) and anatomic structures (ie, Deviation in form, Disk displacement, Displacement of the disc-condyle complex). Seven masticatory muscle disorders were subcategorized into acute and chronic with six conditions being outlined under congenital and developmental disorders.[17]

While referring to the Pertes and Gross classification of TMD, the AACP Guidelines manual sometimes uses a different terminology when designating individual disorders. In addition, the AACP also describes a few conditions not listed by Pertes and Gross (ie, myalgia, trismus, temporal tendinitis, Ernest syndrome) while ignoring others (ie, muscle hypertrophy, myalgia secondary to systemic disease, and all the congenital and developmental disorders).

The AACP classification of TMD has not been subjected to revision since its original publication in 2009. Furthermore, the ICD codes provided are also dated as they originate from the ICD 9th edition. Alternatively, the AACP includes the most common TMD seen in clinics, and the selected TMD categories have relevant labels. However,

Table 1
American Academy of Orofacial Pain taxonomy for temporomandibular disorders[4]

Temporomandibular Joint Disorders
1. Joint pain
   A. Arthralgia [a]
   B. Arthritis [a]
2. Joint disorders
   A. Disk-condyle complex disorders
      i. Disk displacement with reduction
      ii. Disk displacement with reduction with intermittent locking
      iii. Disk displacement without reduction with limited opening
      iv. Disk displacement without reduction without limited opening
   B. Other hypomobility disorders
      i. Adhesions/adherence
      ii. Ankylosis
         a. Fibrous
         b. Osseous
   C. Hypermobility disorders
      i. Subluxation
      ii. Luxation
         a. Closed dislocation
         b. Recurrent dislocation
         c. Ligamentous laxity
3. Joint diseases
   A. Degenerative joint disease
      1. Osteoathrosis
      2. Osteoarthritis [a]
   B. Condylysis
   C. Osteochondritis dissecans
   D. Osteonecrosis
   E. Systemic arthritidis [a]
   F. Neoplasms
   G. Synovial chondromatosis
4. Fracture
   A. Closed fracture of condylar process
   B. Closed fracture of subcondylar process
   C. Open fracture of condylar process
   D. Open fracture of subcondylar process

5. Congenital/developmental disorders
   A. Aplasia
   B. Hypoplasia
   C. Hyperplasia
Masticatory Muscle Disorders
1. Muscle pain
   A. Myalgia [a]
      i. Local myalgia [a]
      ii. Myofascial pain [a]
      iii. Myofascial pain with referral [a]
   B. Tendonitis [a]
   C. Myositis [a]
      i. Noninfective
      ii. Infective
   D. Spasm [a]
2. Contracture
   A. Muscle
   B. Tendon
3. Hypertrophy
4. Neoplasms
   A. Jaw
      i. Malignant
      ii. Benign
   B. Soft tissues of head, face, and neck
      i. Malignant
      ii. Benign
5. Movement disorders
   A. Orofacial dyskinesia
      i. Abnormal involuntary movements
      ii. Ataxia unspecified, muscular incoordination
      iii. Subacute, due to drugs; oral tardive dyskinesia
   B. Oromandibular dystonia
      i. Acute due to drugs
      ii. Deformans, familial, idiopathic, and torsion dystonia
6. Masticatory muscle pain attributed to systemic/central pain disorders
   A. Fibromyalgia[a]
   B. Centrally mediated myalgia[a]
Headache Disorders
1. Headache attributed to TMD [a]
Associated Structures
1. Coronoid hyperplasia

[a] Pain-related TMDs.

the overall scope of TMD is narrower compared with more recent classification schemes, which include subcategories such as joint diseases, neoplasms, and movement disorders. In light of this, the AACP needs to address terminology issues since muscle splinting, trismus, capsulitis, synovitis, and retrodiscitis are no longer used to designate specific TMD as evident in more recent classification systems.

Despite providing expert-driven diagnostic criteria for individual TMD entities, the scope makes the AACP classification less attractive to clinicians.

The International Classification of Orofacial Pain

In 2020 an international collaborative group consisting of members of the OFHP SIG of the IASP, the INfORM group, the AAOP, and the International Headache Society (IHS) published the first edition of the ICOP.[18] This comprehensive hierarchical classification incorporates all types of orofacial pain, including TMD-related pain, with the exception of those not causing pain. Muscle and joint-related painful TMD are grouped into primary and secondary pain disorders under "Myofascial orofacial pain" and "Temporomandibular joint pain." Primary muscle and joint-related pain are subcategorized into acute and chronic using an onset cut-off of greater than 3 months for the later. ICOP uses myofascial orofacial pain as an overarching label for any type of masticatory muscle pain including localized myalgia. Myofascial orofacial pain and temporomandibular joint pain diagnoses can be further subcategorized according to the presence or absence of pain referral during palpation. As previously mentioned, the ICOP (**Table 2**) uses the IASP definition for primary and secondary pain.[10,11]

Okeson Classification of Temporomandibular Disorders (8th Edition)

Okeson's contribution to the classification, diagnosis, and management of TMD has gained significant recognition worldwide through his textbook "Management of Temporomandibular Disorders and Occlusion."[19] Although no organization or association has officially adopted Okeson's classification scheme of TMD, it has nevertheless influenced the evolution and refinement of the current AAOP classification scheme, and many clinicians follow it.

Okeson's TMD classification includes four major groups: (I) Masticatory muscle disorders, (II) temporomandibular joint (TMJ) disorders, (III) Chronic mandibular hypomobility, and (IV) Growth disorders. Except for Group I Masticatory muscle disorders, the other groups have one or more subcategories corresponding to the anatomic structure or underlying pathophysiological process. The proposed comprehensive classification scheme includes 34 individual entities but excludes joint diseases that are not trivial such as condylysis and movement disorders.

Table 2

Taxonomy of pain-related temporomandibular disorders from the International Classification of Orofacial Pain[18]

2. Myofascial orofacial pain
  2.1. Primary myofascial orofacial pain
    2.1.1. Acute primary myofascial orofacial pain
    2.1.2. Chronic primary myofascial orofacial pain
  2.2. Secondary myofascial orofacial pain
    2.2.1. Myofascial orofacial pain attributed to tendonitis
    2.2.2. Myofascial orofacial pain attributed to myositis
    2.2.3. Myofascial orofacial pain attributed to muscle spasm

3. Temporomandibular Joint (TMJ) pain
  3.1. Primary temporomandibular joint pain
    3.1.1. Acute primary temporomandibular joint pain
    3.1.2. Chronic primary temporomandibular joint pain
  3.2. Secondary temporomandibular joint pain
    3.2.1. Temporomandibular joint pain attributed to arthritis
    3.2.2. Temporomandibular joint pain attributed to disk displacement
    3.2.3. Temporomandibular joint pain attributed to degenerative joint disease
    3.2.4. Temporomandibular joint pain attributed to subluxation

DIAGNOSTIC SYSTEMS FOR TEMPOROMANDIBULAR DISORDERS
Research Diagnostic Criteria for Temporomandibular Disorders

In 1992, Dworkin and LeResche[20] published the Research Diagnostic Criteria for Temporomandibular Disorders (RDC/TMD). The aim of this diagnostic system was to provide evidence-based standardized diagnostic criteria for clinical and epidemiologic research purposes. Taking into consideration the biopsychosocial model, the RDC/TMD subdivided the diagnoses into two axes:

- Axis I encompassed clinical diagnoses identifying abnormalities of function and structure of the masticatory muscles or temporomandibular joints.
- Axis II incorporated the assessment of global severity including pain intensity, pain-related disability, depression, and nonspecific physical symptoms.

Over the following decades, these criteria were widely adopted by clinical researchers worldwide and translated into 20 different languages. Research efforts were also conducted to examine and revise the reliability, validity, and clinical utility of the diagnostic system, particularly among the Axis I diagnoses which were based solely on self-report and physical examination.[21–27]

As these diagnostic criteria were not originally intended for clinical practice, only a limited number of subtypes of TMD were included in Axis I (**Box 1**). Hence, these diagnostic categories were broadly defined, for example, the term myofascial pain was used for muscle pain but did not distinguish between local and referred pain. Similarly in Axis II, certain relevant variables to the management of TMD were also omitted from the original publication, such as the assessment of anxiety, sleep disorders, or posttraumatic stress disorder.

Diagnostic Criteria for Temporomandibular Disorders

The International RDC/TMD Consortium of the IADR and the OFHP SIG of the IASP joined forces in 2014 and presented the evidence-based DC/TMD appropriate for both research and clinical settings.[28]

In Axis I, the diagnostic algorithms for the most common TMD were subdivided into pain-related TMD and intra-articular TMD (**Box 2**). A total of 12 diagnoses were included of which all, but myofascial pain and local myalgia, presented specificity and sensitivity data. Less common TMD without demonstrated validity were added to the expanded taxonomic classification (see below).[15]

Box 1
RDC/TMD axis I: clinical TMD conditions[20]

I. Muscle diagnoses
   a. Myofascial pain
   b. Myofascial pain with limited opening

II. Disk displacements
   a. Disk displacement with reduction
   b. Disk displacement without reduction, with limited opening
   c. Disk displacement without reduction, without limited opening

III. Arthralgia, arthritis, arthrosis
   a. Arthralgia
   b. Osteoarthritis of the TMJ
   c. Osteoarthrosis of the TMJ

Box 2
DC/TMD axis I: clinical TMD conditions[20]

Most Common Pain-Related Temporomandibular Disorders
1. Myalgia
   a. Local myalgia
   b. Myofascial pain
   c. Myofascial pain with referral
2. Arthralgia
3. Headache attributed to TMD

Most Common Intra-articular Temporomandibular Disorders
1. Disk displacement with reduction
2. Disk displacement with reduction with intermittent locking
3. Disk displacement without reduction, with limited opening
4. Disk displacement without reduction, without limited opening
5. Degenerative joint disease
6. Subluxation

Axis II was also expanded with the inclusion of a range of assessment tools from screening to a more comprehensive expert evaluation. These new recommendations included a validated TMD pain screener for the identification of pain-related disturbances in any clinical setting.[29] If a patient screen positively, further evaluation for TMD is warranted (**Box 3**).

An important contribution of the DC/TMD was the introduction of criteria that musculoskeletal pains, such as TMD, should be modified (increased or decreased) by function, movement, or parafunction. Moreover, during the clinical examination, provocation tests should reproduce the pain complaint as per the patient's report. The patient should confirm that the provoked pain is *familiar* to their chief complaint.

In addition, in the DC/TMD, the muscle diagnoses were reorganized, and the term myofascial pain in RDC/TMD was replaced by myalgia, which was then subdivided into local myalgia, myofascial pain, and myofascial pain with the referral. Thus, the DC/TMD recognized myofascial pain with referral, as a distinct clinical disorder. For the clinician, understanding pain referral to other anatomic sites, for example, dental structures, is of great relevance in establishing a differential diagnosis and in the consideration of various interventional strategies.

Another update to this diagnostic system was the addition of the diagnosis of "headache attributed to TMD" following the International Classification of Headache Disorders (ICHD). This diagnosis was included in reference to headaches located in the temporalis area modified by jaw function, and the diagnostic criteria showed excellent validity. However, as per ICHD-3 diagnostic classification, the diagnosis of headache attributed to TMD can sometimes overlap the diagnosis of tension-type headache, particularly in patients that present with pericranial tenderness.[30] Although it has some limitations, the DC/TMD remains universally accepted as a reliable diagnostic system for TMD.

Expanded Diagnostic Criteria for Temporomandibular Disorder taxonomy

The expanded taxonomy of the DC/TMD was developed to standardize the diagnosis for the less common TMD that were not included in the DC/TMD structure due to a lack of validated criteria. A total of 37 clinically significant conditions were included by expert consensus. The aim of this expanded diagnostic system of Axis I was to provide a standardized framework for future research studies to investigate the validity of the proposed diagnostic criteria.[15]

Box 3
TMD pain screener[29]

1. In the last 30 days, how long did any pain last in your jaw or temple area on either side?
   a. No pain (0 points)
   b. Pain comes and goes (1 point)
   c. Pain is always present (2 points)

2. In the last 30 days, have you had pain or stiffness in your jaw on awakening?
   a. No (0 points)
   b. Yes (1 point)

3. In the last 30 days, did the following activities change any pain (that is, make it better or make it worse) in your jaw or temple area or on either side?
   A. Chewing hard or tough food
      a. No (0 points)
      b. Yes (1 point)
   B. Opening your mouth or moving your jaw forward or to the side
      a.No (0 points)
      b.Yes (1 point)
   C. Jaw habits such as holding teeth together, clenching, grinding, or chewing gum
      a.No (0 points)
      b.Yes (1 point)
   D. Other jaw activities such as talking, kissing, or yawning
      a. No (0 points)
      b. Yes (1 point)

The three-item version includes questions 1 through 3A, threshold value $\geq$ 2.The six-item version includes questions 1 through 3D, threshold value $\geq$ 3.

International Classification for Orofacial Pain

As previously indicated, the first edition of the ICOP was published in January 2020.[18] As with the DC/TMD, the ICOP classification was intended as a tool to be used for both research and clinical settings. The diagnostic criteria developed for ICOP adopted a similar structure to those present in the ICHD-3 to facilitate its use among different medical specialties dedicated to the diagnosis and management of head and face pain. One of the novel contributions of ICOP in the pain-related TMD category is the consideration of pain frequency. Differentiating between acute and chronic pain is important for the development of better therapeutic interventions as patients suffering from chronic pain are managed differently than acute cases. Interestingly, the ICOP adopted the term myofascial pain to refer to muscle pain, as in the original RDC/TMD nomenclature. Nevertheless, the distinction between local and referred pain was maintained, and specific diagnostic criteria have been proposed for primary chronic myofascial pain with and without a referral. Future research and validity studies will confirm the relevance of the diagnostic subdivisions proposed by the ICOP.

FUTURE DIRECTIONS
Taxonomy Versus Ontology

For classification systems and diagnostic criteria to be relevant and operational, they must follow certain principles and methodologies. Historically, nosologic methodology with taxonomic principles has been implemented.[31] However, this approach is limited by a lack of sensitivity and specificity.[32] An alternative approach following ontological principles has been advocated.[33] Taxonomy assigns a label to the pain condition whereas ontology provides information regarding the pain. However, ontological metrics have limitations as the criteria introduce new terminology that does not have widespread acceptance, are only expert-derived and not evidence-based, and are yet to be tested.[33]

Genetics/Epigenetics

Genetic traits and epigenetic factors involving susceptibility and/or vulnerability to a particular disease and/or treatment response are important factors to consider in TMD patients. This is highlighted by an individual's signs and symptoms as a manifestation of their complex response trait with specific complaints being either amplified or attenuated by their unique genetic makeup and/or prior life experiences.[34] An example of the influence of genetics occurs in relation to the endogenous mu-opioid system.[35] Variations in genotype can result in differences in the synaptic availability of various neurotransmitters such as catecholamines that influence pain perception and brain activation.[36] Past life experiences may alter an individual's adaptive response by modifying the state of the pain-stress response system.[37,38] Furthermore, genetic factors play a role in the etiology of persistent pain conditions by modulating underlying physiologic and psychological processes.[39] Therefore, genetic variants that impact pain sensitivity and psychological traits when combined with environmental factors may interact to influence the risk for the development, initiation, and perpetuation of TMD conditions.[40]

Neurobiological

The incorporation of neurobiological parameters into future classification systems and diagnostic criteria would be beneficial as chronic pain patients experience significant dynamic changes over time.[41–44] This is evidenced by the processes of central neural plasticity as imaging studies have shown alterations in gray-matter volume in chronic pain[45] or as a result of pain relief.[46] The influence of central neural information processing involving learning and memory are now invoked to better explain and describe chronic pain's capability for endurance[47] and how these dimensions exert top-down influences on the rest of physiology.[48]

Biomarkers

A biomarker is a characteristic that can be objectively measured and evaluated as an indicator of a normal biological process, a pathologic process, or pharmacologic (and nonpharmacological) response to a therapeutic intervention.[49] In 2016, a joint FDA-NIH working group (Biomarkers, Endpoints, and other Tools – BEST) identified seven distinct biomarker categories that could be applied across the whole spectrum of biological research.[50] Candidate biomarkers and potential applicable tests that should be considered can be categorized by physiologic tests, psychological or behavioral characteristics, use of imaging, and molecular and protein assays.[51] Each one of these modalities has supporting evidence as being used either clinically and/or experimentally for the diagnosis, measurement of burden of disease, or determination of the prognosis or efficacy of treatment of pain conditions.[51] Unfortunately, the current landscape for using the predictive value of available biomarkers in diagnosing pain is rather low[51] despite efforts of ongoing research.[40,52] It is also unfortunate that other diagnostic aids, be it laboratory and/or imaging studies, are also largely only research based.[39,53,54] Therefore, the current state of diagnosis remains heavily reliant on patient self-report making diagnosis of pain conditions as much an art form as a pure science.[32]

Precision Medicine

Precision medicine, using a P4 approach, incorporates the following: prediction, prevention, personalization, and participation.[55] Prediction relates to identifying the genetic risks for diseases with signs of illness recognized before its manifestation. Prevention involves in providing the individual with the tools to recognize the earliest signs of the disease when it is most reversible. Personalization focuses on the individualization and optimization of wellness by predicting disease and designing personalized interventions for management. Participation facilitates that the individual should be well informed about their health and better prepared to make their own health care decisions. Incorporating the P4 approach into TMD classification systems and diagnostic criteria will pave the way for enhanced patient care.

Artificial Intelligence

Artificial intelligence (AI) consists of developing computational systems that can perform human intelligence tasks to assist with decision-making support.[49] AI, due to its ability to accumulate, analyze and draw inferences from vast amounts of data is providing a paradigm shift toward precision medicine.[56] Within AI is the concept of machine learning (ML), the process of developing algorithms with the ability to learn without being explicitly programmed. This approach removes the "expert" brain from making an interpretation from the accumulated data.[49] A subset of ML is deep learning that involves artificial neural networks adapting and learning from vast amounts of collected data. AI methods and ML algorithms will allow for the phenotyping, endotyping, and the selection of management strategies for TMD. This process will transform the role of practitioners to be the translator of the technical data for the patient, act as a guide in assisting the patient in understanding their digital health and be a counselor in navigating through health care choices.[57]

In summary, the future is very bright for developing more precise and accurate classification and diagnostic systems. By incorporating ontological principles involving the use of genetic traits/epigenetic factors and following neurobiological principles with biomarkers in addition to the assistance afforded by AI, the potential for following precision medicine involving pain conditions is within our grasp.

CLINICS CARE POINTS

- Current classification systems for TMD are essential for providing a framework of information that allow the provision of quality diagnosis and enhanced patient management. It is important to recognize these systems need to evolve in order to provide greater patient targeted care.

- Currently, there is a lack of a unique and universal classification of TMD, however, the classification scheme proposed by the American Academy of Orofacial Pain (AAOP) can be currently used as a best practices model.

- The current version of the Diagnostic Criteria for Temporomandibular Disorders (DC/TMD) can be used both for clinical and research purposes as a universally accepted reliable evidence-based diagnostic system for common temporomandibular disorders.

- The integration and incorporation of ontological principles, genetics /epigenetics vulnerability factors, neurobiological processes and biomarkers, the concepts of precision medicine and the application of artificial intelligence will ultimately coalesce and result in a treatment oriented classification system for TMD.

DISCLOSURE

The authors have nothing to disclose.

REFERENCES

1. Merriam-Webster. Definition of classification. 2022. Available at: http://www.merriam-webster.com/dictionary/classification. Accessed April 16, 2022.
2. Felson DT, Anderson JJ. Methodological and statistical approaches to criteria development in rheumatic diseases. Baillieres Clin Rheumatol 1995;9:253–66.
3. Fillingim RB, Bruehl S, Dworkin RH, et al. The ACTTION-american pain society pain taxonomy (AAPT): an evidence-based and multidimensional approach to classifying chronic pain conditions. J Pain 2014;15:241–9.
4. De Leeuw R, Klasser GD. Orofacial pain: guidelines for assessment, diagnosis, and management. 6th edition. Chicago: Quintessence; 2018.
5. Naeije M, Te Veldhuis AH, Te Veldhuis EC, et al. Disc displacement within the human temporomandibular joint: a systematic review of a 'noisy annoyance'. J Oral Rehabil 2013;40:139–58.
6. Aggarwal R, Ringold S, Khanna D, et al. Distinctions between diagnostic and classification criteria? Arthritis Care Res (Hoboken) 2015;67:891–7.
7. June RR, Aggarwal R. The use and abuse of diagnostic/classification criteria. Best Pract Res Clin Rheumatol 2014;28:921–34.
8. International classification of diseases 11th revision. 2022. Available at: https://icd.who.int/browse11/l-m/en. Accessed April 10, 2022.
9. Treede RD, Rief W, Barke A, et al. Chronic pain as a symptom or a disease: the IASP Classification of Chronic Pain for the International Classification of Diseases (ICD-11). Pain 2019;160:19–27.
10. Nicholas M, Vlaeyen JWS, Rief W, et al. The IASP classification of chronic pain for ICD-11: chronic primary pain. Pain 2019;160:28–37.
11. Benoliel R, Svensson P, Evers S, et al. The IASP classification of chronic pain for ICD-11: chronic secondary headache or orofacial pain. Pain 2019;160:60–8.
12. Arnold LM, Bennett RM, Crofford LJ, et al. AAPT Diagnostic criteria for fibromyalgia. J Pain 2019;20:611–28.
13. Freeman R, Edwards R, Baron R, et al. AAPT diagnostic criteria for peripheral neuropathic pain: focal and segmental disorders. J Pain 2019;20:369–93.
14. Kent ML, Tighe PJ, Belfer I, et al. The ACTTION-APS-AAPM pain taxonomy (AAAPT) multidimensional approach to classifying acute pain conditions. J Pain 2017;18:479–89.
15. Peck CC, Goulet JP, Lobbezoo F, et al. Expanding the taxonomy of the diagnostic criteria for temporomandibular disorders. J Oral Rehabil 2014;41:2–23.
16. American Academy of Craniofacial Pain. Craniofacial pain: a handbook for assessment, diagnosis and management. Chattanooga: Chroma, Inc.; 2009.
17. Pertes RA, Gross SG. Clinical management of temporomandibular disorders and orofacial pain. Chicago: Quintessence Books; 1995.
18. International classification of orofacial pain, 1st edition (ICOP). Cephalalgia 2020;40:129–221.
19. Okeson JP. Management of temporomandibular disorders and occlusion. 8th edition. St. Louis: Mosby; 2019.
20. Dworkin SF, LeResche L. Research diagnostic criteria for temporomandibular disorders: review, criteria, examinations and specifications, critique. J Craniomandib Disord 1992;6:301–55.
21. Schiffman EL, Truelove EL, Ohrbach R, et al. The research diagnostic criteria for temporomandibular disorders. i: overview and methodology for assessment of validity. J Orofac Pain 2010;24:7–24.

22. Look JO, John MT, Tai F, et al. The research diagnostic criteria for temporomandibular disorders. iI: reliability of Axis I diagnoses and selected clinical measures. J Orofac Pain 2010;24:25–34.

23. Truelove E, Pan W, Look JO, et al. The research diagnostic criteria for temporomandibular disorders. iii: validity of Axis I diagnoses. J Orofac Pain 2010;24: 35–47.

24. Ohrbach R, Turner JA, Sherman JJ, et al. The research diagnostic criteria for temporomandibular disorders. iv: evaluation of psychometric properties of the axis ii measures. J Orofac Pain 2010;24:48–62.

25. Schiffman EL, Ohrbach R, Truelove EL, et al. The research diagnostic criteria for temporomandibular disorders. v: methods used to establish and validate revised Axis I diagnostic algorithms. J Orofac Pain 2010;24:63–78.

26. Anderson GC, Gonzalez YM, Ohrbach R, et al. The research diagnostic criteria for temporomandibular disorders. vi: future directions. J Orofac Pain 2010;24: 79–88.

27. Dworkin SF. Research diagnostic criteria for temporomandibular disorders: current status & future relevance. J Oral Rehabil 2010;37:734–43.

28. Schiffman E, Ohrbach R, Truelove E, et al. Diagnostic criteria for temporomandibular disorders (DC/TMD) for clinical and research applications: recommendations of the international RDC/TMD consortium network* and orofacial pain special interest. J Oral Facial Pain Headache 2014;28:6–27.

29. Gonzalez YM, Schiffman E, Gordon SM, et al. Development of a brief and effective temporomandibular disorder pain screening questionnaire: reliability and validity. J Am Dent Assoc 2011;142:1183–91.

30. Headache Classification Committee of the International Headache Society (IHS). The international classification of headache disorders, 3rd edition (ICHD-3). Cephalalgia 2018;38:1–211.

31. Raj P. Taxonomy and classification of pain. In: Kreitler S, Beltrutti D, Lamberto A, et al, editors. The handbook of chronic pain. New York: Nova Biomedical Books by Nova Science Publishers; 2007. p. 41–56.

32. Ceusters W, Michelotti A, Raphael KG, et al. Perspectives on next steps in classification of oro-facial pain - part 1: role of ontology. J Oral Rehabil 2015;42: 926–41.

33. Nixdorf DR, Drangsholt MT, Ettlin DA, et al. Classifying orofacial pains: a new proposal of taxonomy based on ontology. J Oral Rehabil 2012;39:161–9.

34. Stohler CS. Taking stock: from chasing occlusal contacts to vulnerability alleles. Orthod Craniofac Res 2004;7:157–61.

35. Zubieta JK, Smith YR, Bueller JA, et al. Regional mu opioid receptor regulation of sensory and affective dimensions of pain. Science 2001;293:311–5.

36. Zubieta JK, Heitzeg MM, Smith YR, et al. COMT val158met genotype affects mu-opioid neurotransmitter responses to a pain stressor. Science 2003;299:1240–3.

37. Gupta A, Silman AJ, Ray D, et al. The role of psychosocial factors in predicting the onset of chronic widespread pain: results from a prospective population-based study. Rheumatology (Oxford) 2007;46:666–71.

38. Slavich GM, Tartter MA, Brennan PA, et al. Endogenous opioid system influences depressive reactions to socially painful targeted rejection life events. Psychoneuroendocrinology 2014;49:141–9.

39. Smith SB, Maixner DW, Greenspan JD, et al. Potential genetic risk factors for chronic TMD: genetic associations from the OPPERA case control study. J Pain 2011;12(11 Suppl):T92–101.

40. Maixner W, Diatchenko L, Dubner R, et al. Orofacial pain prospective evaluation and risk assessment study–the OPPERA study. J Pain 2011;12(11 Suppl): T4–11, e1-2.
41. Diatchenko L, Nackley AG, Slade GD, et al. Idiopathic pain disorders–pathways of vulnerability. Pain 2006;123:226–30.
42. Apkarian AV, Baliki MN, Farmer MA. Predicting transition to chronic pain. Curr Opin Neurol 2013;26:360–7.
43. Bourne S, Machado AG, Nagel SJ. Basic anatomy and physiology of pain pathways. Neurosurg Clin N Am 2014;25:629–38.
44. Borsook D, Youssef AM, Simons L, et al. When pain gets stuck: the evolution of pain chronification and treatment resistance. Pain 2018;159:2421–36.
45. Smallwood RF, Laird AR, Ramage AE, et al. Structural brain anomalies and chronic pain: a quantitative meta-analysis of gray matter volume. J Pain 2013; 14:663–75.
46. Borsook D, Erpelding N, Becerra L. Losses and gains: chronic pain and altered brain morphology. Expert Rev Neurother 2013;13:1221–34.
47. Price TJ, Inyang KE. Commonalities between pain and memory mechanisms and their meaning for understanding chronic pain. Prog Mol Biol Transl Sci 2015;131: 409–34.
48. Reichling DB, Levine JD. Critical role of nociceptor plasticity in chronic pain. Trends Neurosci 2009;32:611–8.
49. Tracey I, Woolf CJ, Andrews NA. Composite pain biomarker signatures for objective assessment and effective treatment. Neuron 2019;101:783–800.
50. FDA-NIH Biomarker Working Group. BEST (biomarkers, EndpointS and other tools) resource. Bethesda (MD): Silver Spring, National Institutes of Health (US); 2016.
51. Ceusters W, Nasri-Heir C, Alnaas D, et al. Perspectives on next steps in classification of oro-facial pain - Part 3: biomarkers of chronic oro-facial pain - from research to clinic. J Oral Rehabil 2015;42:956–66.
52. Fillingim RB, Slade GD, Diatchenko L, et al. Summary of findings from the OPPERA baseline case-control study: implications and future directions. J Pain 2011;12(11 Suppl):T102–7.
53. Maixner W, Greenspan JD, Dubner R, et al. Potential autonomic risk factors for chronic TMD: descriptive data and empirically identified domains from the OPPERA case-control study. J Pain 2011;12(11 Suppl):T75–91.
54. Slade GD, Conrad MS, Diatchenko L, et al. Cytokine biomarkers and chronic pain: association of genes, transcription, and circulating proteins with temporomandibular disorders and widespread palpation tenderness. Pain 2011;152: 2802–12.
55. Hood L, Flores M. A personal view on systems medicine and the emergence of proactive P4 medicine: predictive, preventive, personalized and participatory. N Biotechnol 2012;29:613–24.
56. Johnson KB, Wei WQ, Weeraratne D, et al. Precision medicine, ai, and the future of personalized health care. Clin Transl Sci 2021;14:86–93.
57. Mesko B. The real era of the art of medicine begins with artificial intelligence. J Med Internet Res 2019;21:e16295.

Temporomandibular Joint Imaging

Steven R. Singer, DDS[a],*, Mel Mupparapu, DMD, MDS, Dipl ABOMR[b]

KEYWORDS

- Imaging • TMJ • Panoramic • Cone-beam computed tomography • MRI
- Arthrography

KEY POINTS

- Radiographic examinations are individually prescribed.
- Imaging is selected based on complaint, anamnesis, and clinical findings.
- There is no single ideal imaging study for temporomandibular disorders (TMDs).
- Oral and maxillofacial radiologists can aid in reaching an accurate diagnosis of TMDs.

INTRODUCTION

The temporomandibular joints (TMJs) form the articulation between the cranium and the mandible. The osseous components include the mandibular condyles and the temporal bones. The articulation consists of two synovial joints, which enclose articular discs of dense, fibrous, connective tissue. They are classified as a hinge joint with a movable socket.

The first and foremost question that should be answered is "Why are we imaging this anatomy?" In general, we image to confirm clinically suspected disorders, disease, and other pathologic entities. Further, properly selected imaging can yield information such as the location and type of lesion, extent of change to the normal structures, and ultimately lead to improved management of disease.

Basic rules of radiographic selection criteria apply to TMJ imaging. Radiographs, as well as nonionizing radiation-based imaging examinations, are selected based on patient complaint and history, findings from clinical examination, and patient's medical history. Once this information is gathered, a clinical diagnosis is formulated, and an imaging study may be prescribed. Because the TMJ is composed of both calcified and noncalcified tissues, each type of tissue needs its own specialized imaging.

---

[a] Department of Diagnostic Sciences, Rutgers School of Dental Medicine, 110 Bergen Street, Room D885A, Newark, NJ 07103-2400, USA; [b] University of Pennsylvania School of Dental Medicine, Philadelphia, PA, USA
* Corresponding author.
E-mail address: singerst@sdm.rutgers.edu

Dent Clin N Am 67 (2023) 227–241
https://doi.org/10.1016/j.cden.2022.11.001
0011-8532/23/© 2022 Elsevier Inc. All rights reserved.

Further, radiation safety, including concepts such as ALARA (as low as reasonably achievable) and ALADA-IP (as low as diagnostically acceptable being indication-oriented and patient-specific)[1,2] should be applied. In general, imaging studies should be limited to region of interest (ROI) and use the lowest dose of ionizing radiation possible, based on the available equipment. For example, many newer panoramic machines can provide excellent quality four-view TMJ studies while limiting exposure to other regions of the orofacial structures. In the same vein, limited field of view (FOV) cone-beam computed tomography (CBCT) scans should be considered rather than large FOV scans. Because CBCT examinations deliver a higher dose of ionizing radiation to the patient, the potential benefit versus potential harm needs to be more carefully examined.

Imaging modalities that are used in TMJ studies include panoramic imaging, plain film, arthrography, computed tomography, and MRI.

It should be stated that the prescriber is responsible for interpretation of the entire imaging study and not just the ROI. MRI studies are typically done at imaging centers and the attending radiologist will return the study with a report, whereas reporting in-office imaging studies are the responsibility of the prescriber. Oral and maxillofacial radiologists are able to assist in providing radiology reports for panoramic, CBCT, MRI, and other imaging studies of the TMJs.[3]

The most common disabling condition affecting the TMJ is rheumatoid arthritis (RA). Based on the American College of Rheumatology/European League Against Rheumatism criteria for the diagnosis of RA.[4] TMJ RA diagnosis in the absence of any other joint involvement in the body can only be made if it is bilateral and the following criteria are met:

1. Abnormal C-reactive protein and erythrocyte sedimentation rates
2. Low-positive or high-positive rheumatoid factor and anticitrullinated protein antibodies
3. Duration of symptoms is approximately six weeks or greater.

The radiographic diagnosis forms a key role in the assessment of TMJ RA (**Figs. 1** and **2**). TMJ is involved in approximately 50% of cases with rheumatoid diseases such as RA, ankylosing spondylitis, and psoriatic arthritis.[4–8]

Imaging the TMJ allows clinicians to evaluate the integrity and relationships of the TMJ osseous components and soft tissue. The choice of TMJ imaging depends on several factors such as radiation dose, cost, availability, diagnostic information provided, and whether hard or soft tissue is imaged.[8] When diagnosing TMD, hard tissues

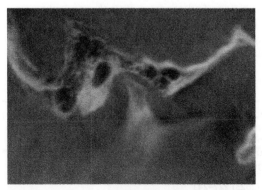

Fig. 1. CBCT adjusted sagittal projection of the right TMJ demonstrating significant erosive changes to the mandibular condyle, glenoid fossa, and articular eminence secondary to RA.

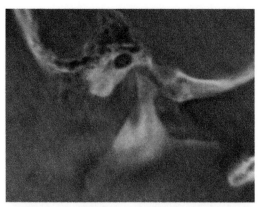

Fig. 2. CBCT adjusted sagittal projection of the left TMJ demonstrating significant erosive changes to the mandibular condyle, glenoid fossa, and articular eminence secondary to RA.

are the first to be evaluated. Osseous contours, positional relationship of the condyle and glenoid fossa and range of motion are assessed.[5] Soft tissue imaging offers information about disk position and morphology, as well as abnormalities surrounding the muscle and soft tissue.[9]

PANORAMIC IMAGING

Panoramic images are curved surface tomograms. They provide broad coverage of the orofacial structures at a relatively low dose of ionizing radiation and a minimum of discomfort for the patient. Although there is variation based on the specifics of the imaging systems used, it is reported that the effective dose for a single periapical radiograph is approximately 0.001 and 0.007 mSv for a standard panoramic radiograph.[10] The dose for a four-view TMJ tomographic images may be lower (**Figs. 3 and 4**). Panoramic imaging of the joints allows for sagittal projections of the joints with an adequate resolution for detecting anatomic changes as may be seen in degenerative joint diseases such as osteoarthritis and RA or anatomic variants such as bifid condyle, as well as fractures (**Fig. 5**). With proper splinting and patient positioning, condylar position in the glenoid fossa and along the articular eminence, dislocations, hypermobility, and changes in joint space can be seen on a qualitative basis. Panoramic radiographs, used along with reverse Towne's views, can provide excellent imaging of condylar fractures.

Inaccuracies in the measurable distance are a limitation of the panoramic technique. Caution is recommended in making absolute measurements using panoramic radiographs.[11]

PLANAR IMAGING (PLAIN IMAGING OR 2D IMAGING)

Due to compression and superimposition of the z-axis, most plain film views, such as lateral and posteroanterior cephalometric and skull projections, are of limited use in TMJ diagnosis. Exceptions are reverse Towne's views, as well as transcranial, transorbital, and transpharyngeal images. Although CBCT has superseded these imaging modalities, CBCT or multidetector computed tomography (MDCT) imaging is not always easily accessible.

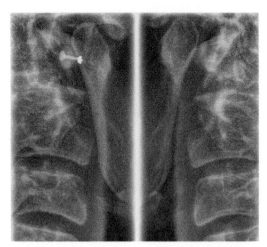

Fig. 3. TMJ tomographic view in closed mouth position. Typically, these tomographic projections are used to check the range of motion of the condyles as well as the anatomical variations and pathologic condition within the joint. If there is a disc-related disorder, MR imaging of the joint will be needed to evaluate the disc position and morphology.

Reverse Towne's projections are posteroanterior views taken with the patient's chin tilted downward and the mouth in an open position, providing a clear view of the condylar neck and a portion of the condylar head. As mentioned earlier, along with a panoramic image, the reverse Towne's view can allow viewing of subcondylar fractures.

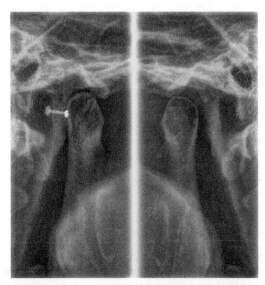

Fig. 4. TMJ tomographic view in open mouth position. Typically, these tomographic projections are used to check the range of motion of the condyles as well as the anatomical variations and pathologic condition within the joint. If there is a disc-related disorder, MR imaging of the joint will be needed to evaluate the disc position and morphology.

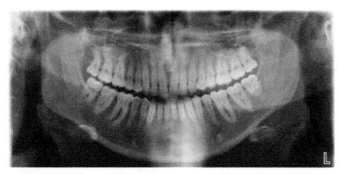

Fig. 5. Panoramic projection demonstrating fracture of the left condylar neck. Note the entire glenoid fossa is not covered in this radiograph due to positioning issues related to the patient after the trauma.

Transcranial and transpharyngeal projections provide adjusted sagittal projections of the TMJs. They may be taken in both the open and closed positions, with stenting recommended for consistent open position views. These views are technically challenging, as care must be taken in positioning to avoid superimposition of the petrous ridge of the temporal bone over the joint. Transorbital projections provide adjusted coronal projections of the TMJ, allowing for visualization of medio-lateral changes to the condylar head and glenoid fossa.

Although these extraoral plain film views have been all but replaced by CBCT, a 2019 study comparing the efficacy of transcranial views to CT imaging in the diagnosis of osteoarthritis and RA found that both methods "are equally efficacious in evaluating the osseous degenerative changes of TMJ in arthritis."[12]

LINEAR AND PLURIDIRECTIONAL TOMOGRAPHY

Tomography (from Greek, meaning "picture of a slice") uses motion to blur structures that are located in front or in back of the ROI. This is especially helpful in projectional imaging of the skull base, where many bony structures are in close proximity. Linear tomography was developed initially but proved to be of questionable value due to strong streaking artifacts created by structures outside of the image layer. These artifacts were often superimposed over the ROI, rendering the imaging of little value. During the 1990s, pluridirectional tomography systems, designed for orofacial imaging, were developed. These provided higher quality images than linear tomography but required a large amount of time for each study. They were ultimately retired when CBCT image became more available.

Arthrography and Arthrocentesis

Arthrography is a technique where a radiopaque dye is injected into a joint and then the joint is imaged. It has been used for TMJ imaging to determine if a disc is displaced or perforated. Arthrography provides an indirect depiction of the disc because the dye will be seen in the inferior joint space beneath the disc and in the superior joint space above the disc. Great care must be taken to inject the proper amount of dye so as to enter the joint spaces while not overwhelming the joint and obscuring the anatomic structures. Arthrography can be used to depict the anterior–posterior relationship of the disc, perforation, and joint function, when open and closed images are exposed.

It is considered to be inaccurate for medial and lateral displacement. Arthrography is considered to be extremely technique sensitive.

Traditionally, the images were obtained following introduction of the dye into the joint using plain film techniques, including transcranial and transpharyngeal projections. More recently, CBCT imaging has been used, providing three-dimensional arthrography of the TMJ. The researchers were able to use the images to diagnose disc displacement, both with and without reduction, disc perforation, and tears in the articular capsule.[13]

Computed Tomography

Although MDCT may be used for TMJ imaging of both the hard and soft tissues, its use in recent years has been superseded by CBCT for hard tissue imaging and MRI for visualizing the soft tissues of the joint. CBCT has demonstrated its superiority over MDCT for TMJ imaging through its high-quality images of the hard tissues of the TMJ, versatile software that permits oblique views to accommodate the variable angles of the joint, increasing accessibility in dental practices, small FOV scans that may reduce artifact production, and significantly lower radiation dose. Thin cross-sections of the joint may be obtained, and the resolution is usually adequate for diagnosis. Further, three-dimensional reconstructions are easily viewed and may be rotated.

CBCT is able to reliably demonstrate the hard tissue changes commonly seen in patients with degenerative changes to the joint. These changes include remodeling of the articulating surface of the condylar head, osteophyte formation, subchondral cysts, osteosclerosis, and remodeling of the posterior slope of the articular eminence (**Figs. 6** and **7**). **Fig. 8** is a CBCT 3-D reconstruction of right TMJ showing significant condylar erosion and morphological changes.

Further findings that are often seen on CBCT examinations include bifid condyles (**Fig. 9**) and reduced joint space—a possible indirect indicator of disc displacement. Condylar fractures are also nicely demonstrated in coronal and axial projections (**Figs. 10** and **11**). **Figs. 12** and **13** show sagittal and coronal projections of a separated osteophyte in the superior joint space of the right TMJ. Ankylosis of the TMJs can also be viewed using CBCT scans, especially if the ankylosis is bony (**Figs. 14–16**).

Most CBCT software programs allow for a "TMJ View." This feature proves adjusted sagittal slices at a variable angle for each joint. Axial and coronal views of the joints are also provided (see **Fig. 14**; **Fig. 17**).

Magnetic Resonance Imaging

When imaging of the soft tissues of the TMJ is required, MRI provides the only viable option for visualization of the articular disc.[14] MRI is based on nonionizing radiation but does have some absolute and relative contraindications. MRI yields fewer artifacts from dense bone and metallic structures. It is accurate for both soft and hard tissues. Timing of the radiofrequency pulses alters the appearance of the images. Although there are several sequences available, T1-weighted (T1W) and T2W images are still used most frequently for MR imaging of the TMJs.[14] T1W imaging provides a bright signal for fat, whereas T2W imaging yields images where both fat and water appear bright. The contrast of the tissues in the image is, in general, based on the water content of the tissue. The higher the water content, the brighter the signal in the resultant image. Therefore, dense bone (low water content) will usually appear black in an MRI, whereas fluids, such as fat, will appear brighter. In the images of the TMJ, the articular disc will appear dark gray because it is composed of dense fibrous connective tissue with a low water content. The retrodiscal tissue will appear brighter. T1W images

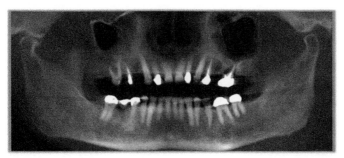

Fig. 6. CBCT-based panoramic reconstruction showing significant TMJ changes within the right condyle.

provide excellent contrast resolution of soft tissues, displaying a wide range of intermediate gray densities that allow for visualization of the various tissues that comprise the TMJs. T2W imaging is prescribed when fluid accumulation is suspected. This might be in cases of joint effusion, osteonecrosis, or cystic lesions.

Absolute contraindications to MRI include cerebral aneurysm clips and cardiac pacemakers. Relative contraindications are claustrophobia, metallic prosthetic heart valves, ferromagnetic bodies, and implanted wires in critical locations. Surgical clips outside of the brain and other nonferrous metal prostheses are not contraindications to MRI. Additionally, dental implants that are made of titanium, zirconium, or other nonferrous substances are not contraindications to MRI. If there is any doubt, consultation with the patient's physician to clarify the nature of the implanted device is appropriate. MRI is limited by relatively low resolution. When high-resolution MR imaging is required, the prescriber should request that a minimum of a 1.5 Tesla scanner be

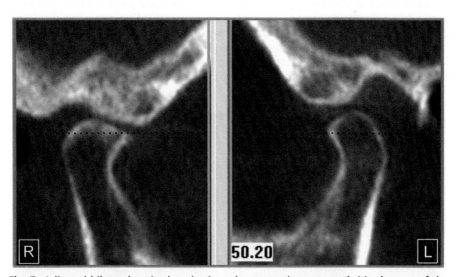

Fig. 7. Adjusted bilateral sagittal projections demonstrating osteoarthritic changes of the TMJs. Flattening of the anterior articulating surfaces of the condylar head and osteophyte formation are seen in both joints, whereas more advanced degenerative changes, including flattening of the posterior slope of the articular eminence, reduced joint space, and subchondral cyst formation, are noted in the right TMJ.

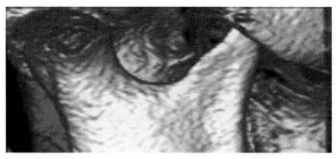

Fig. 8. CBCT 3-D reconstruction of right TMJ showing significant condylar erosion and morphological changes.

used. Tesla is a derived SI unit of magnetic field strength. Higher Tesla scanners will provide improved resolution.

Indications for MRI of the TMJs include suspected displacements, joint effusion following trauma, osteomyelitis of the condylar head and/or articular eminence, and neoplasia. Although functional MRI[15] is not yet readily available, open and closed MRI studies are often appropriate to distinguish between disc displacement with and without reduction (**Figs. 18** and **19**).

Ultrasound Imaging

Ultrasound (US) imaging is an inexpensive and noninvasive diagnostic imaging modality that is widely available. US imaging has high sensitivity for disc evaluation, cartilage displacement, joint effusion, and condylar erosion.[16,17] However, MR diagnosis of TMD is preferred over US diagnosis by clinicians due to its higher specificity. Limitations in the use of US include image distortion and variability in the interpretation of image data. US imaging can be used for the evaluation of TMD but it does not provide definitive diagnoses. Due to the nature of the US frequencies, only the osseous surfaces but not the cortex or spongiosa can be visualized. There is limited accessibility of deep structures by US evaluation due to the absorption of sound waves by the lateral portions of condyles and the zygomatic process of the temporal bone.

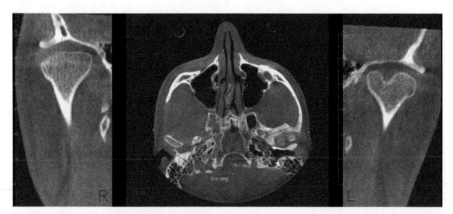

Fig. 9. CBCT coronal and axial projections of the TMJs. Left side exhibits bifid nature of the condyle. The right condyle is unremarkable.

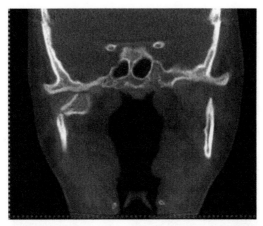

Fig. 10. CBCT coronal projection at the level of the condyles demonstrating a right subcondylar fracture.

Nuclear Imaging (Bone Scanning and Positron Emission Scanning)

Nuclear medicine scans can be used for the evaluation of osseous pathologic conditions in the TMJ. Technetium-99 m bone scans are the most commonly used scintigraphic studies. Technetium bone scans have relatively high resolution and high sensitivity. Radiation exposure and lack of specificity are the drawbacks. Advantages include low cost and high diagnostic accuracy for osseous pathologic conditions. Bone scans are best suited for assessing the progress of TMD, especially the inflammatory conditions and/or remodeling of TMJ. This is especially true in the prediction of painful temporomandibular joint osteoarthritis in juvenile patients.[18]

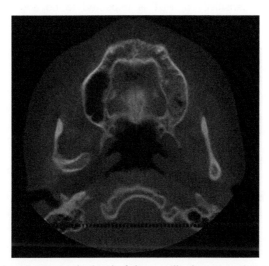

Fig. 11. CBCT axial projection at the level of the maxilla demonstrating a right subcondylar fracture.

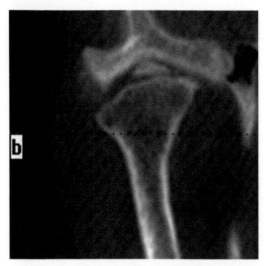

Fig. 12. CBCT coronal projection of the right TMJ. In addition to the osteoarthritic changes seen in the joint, a separated osteophyte is seen in the superior joint space.

Inflammation of the TMJ has a high correlation to the late stages of RA. TMJ is the freely moving joint between the condyle of the mandible and the squamous portion of the temporal bone. The TMJ consists of six main parts: the ligaments, the lateral pterygoid, the articular disc, the capsule, the articular surface to the temporal bone and the mandibular condyles. Most of these structures can be seen by CT scans. Imaging the TMJ using positron emission scanning (PET) is a new development. TMJ disorders are generally diagnosed using full-skull radiograph, MRI, CBCT, or CT as describe earlier in this article. MRI can demonstrate position of the articular disc (see **Figs. 18** and **19**) and CT demonstrates the osseous detail of the joint. PET, however, can show not only the bony structures but also soft tissue inflammation, as well as the impact on blood flow (**Fig. 20**). The sensitivity of PET is expected to be a great advantage for

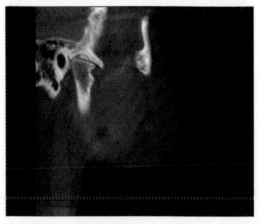

Fig. 13. CBCT sagittal projection of the right TMJ. In addition to the osteoarthritic changes seen in the joint, a separated osteophyte is seen in the superior joint space.

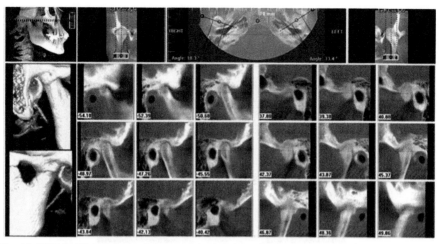

Fig. 14. TMJ CBCT. Ankylosis of the condylar heads to the posterior wall of the glenoid fossa can be seen bilaterally. This condition is the result of RA.

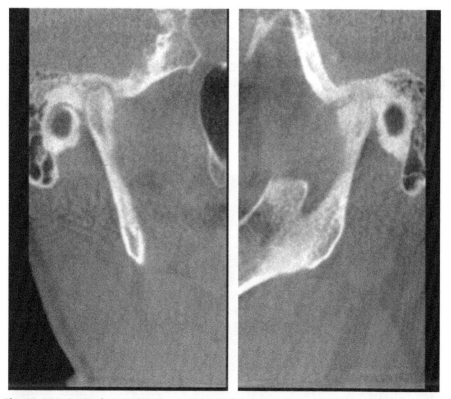

Fig. 15. TMJ Sagittal CBCT showing ankylosis of the condylar heads to the posterior wall of the glenoid fossa seen bilaterally. This condition is the result of RA.

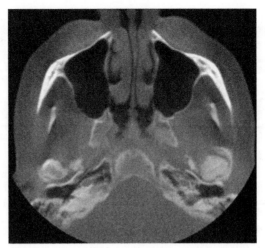

Fig. 16. TMJ axial CBCT at the level of the condyles showing the bilateral ankylosis. This condition is the result of RA.

diagnosing TMD. Both [18F]-fluoro-2-deoxy-D-glucose (FDG) and [18F]-sodium fluoride (NaF) are used in the diagnosis of inflammatory disorders of TMJ. FDG is an analog of glucose that contains the radionuclide, Fluorine F-18, which decays by positron emission. Its efficacy comes from the optimal half-life and low degradability. Dr Abass Alavi conducted the first human study with FGD-PET in 1976 leading to a breakthrough in nuclear medicine.[19] FDG-PET/CT and NaF-PET/CT have high TMJ uptake in patients with RA. Overall, both FDG-PET/CT and NaF-PET/CT are reliable imaging tools that can be helpful in a clinical setting for patients with TMD.

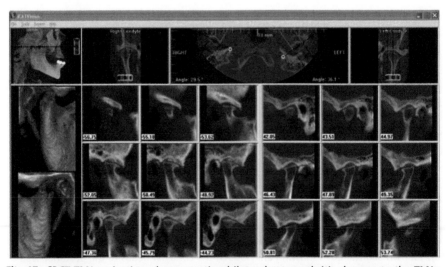

Fig. 17. CBCT TMJ projections demonstrating bilateral osteoarthritic changes to the TMJs.

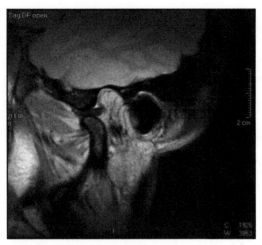

Fig. 18. T1W MRI of the joint (open mouth) demonstrating normal disc position although disc itself has some morphological changes.

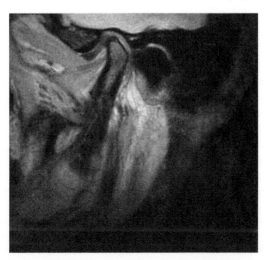

Fig. 19. T1W MRI of the joint (closed mouth) demonstrating anterior disc displacement.

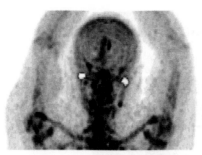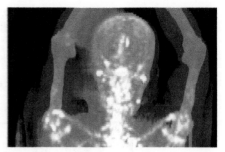

Fig. 20. PET maximum intensity projections. The lit-up areas in color indicate TMJ increased metabolic activity in a patient with rheumatoid arthritis. (Images courtesy Sophia Oak, Temple University, Philadelphia, PA).

SUMMARY

Diagnostic imaging of the temporomandibular joint can provide confirmation of clinically suspected temporomandibular disorders. Careful selection of the imaging examination with respect to the tissues being imaged and the radiation burden to the patient will aid in obtaining the desired diagnostic yield. In general, ionizing radiation-based imaging is most appropriate for hard tissue abnormalities, whereas MRI is indicated for soft tissue pathologic conditions and anatomic variations.

CLINICS CARE POINTS

- Select imaging studies based on supected conditions.
- Consider the suspected anatomic changes and match the imaging study that is best suited to visualize these changes.
- The practitioner is responsible for complete interpretation of the prescribed images.
- Consider the potential risk to the patient versus the potential benefit of the imaging study.

DISCLOSURE

S.R. Singer has nothing to disclose. M. Mupparapu has nothing to disclose.

REFERENCES

1. Oenning AC, Jacobs R, Pauwels R, et al, DIMITRA Research Group. Cone-beam CT in paediatric dentistry: DIMITRA project position statement. Pediatr Radiol 2018;48(3):308–16. Available at: http://www.dimitra.be.
2. Oenning AC, Jacobs R, Salmon B, DIMITRA Research Group. ALADAIP, beyond ALARA and towards personalized optimization for paediatric cone-beam CT. Int J Paediatr Dent 2021;31(5):676–8. Available at: http://www.dimitra.be.
3. Kim IH, Singer SR, Mupparapu M. Review of cone beam computed tomography guidelines in North America. Quintessence Int 2019;50(2):136–45.
4. Som PM, Curtin HD. Head and neck imaging. 5th edition. St Louis (MO): Elsevier Mosby; 2004. p. 1598f.

5. Glupker L, Kula K, Parks E, et al. Three-dimensional computed tomography analysis of airway volume changes between open and closed jaw positions. Am J Orthod Dentofacial Orthop 2015;147(4):426–34.
6. Gruber A, McCullogh J, Sidebottom AJ. Medium-term outcomes and complications after total replacement of the temporomandibular joint. Prospective outcome analysis after 3 and 5 years. Br J Oral Maxillofac Surg 2015;53:412–5.
7. Ruparelia PB, Shah DS, Ruparelia K, et al. Bilateral TMJ involvement in rheumatoid arthritis. Case Rep Dent 2014;2014:262430.
8. Ahmed N, Mustafa HM, Catrina AI, et al. Impact of temporomandibular joint pain in rheumatoid arthritis. Mediators Inflamm 2013;2013:587419.
9. Koenig LJ (Editor). Tamimi D, Petrikowski CG, Harnsberger HR, Ruprecht A, Benson BW et al. Diagnostic Imaging. Oral and maxilofacial. 1st ed. Amirsys. Salt Lake City, U: 2012.
10. Jenkins WM, Brocklebank LM, Winning SM, et al. A comparison of two radiographic assessment protocols for patients with periodontal disease. Br Dent J 2005;198(9):565–9 [discussion: 557]; [quiz: 586].
11. Laster WS, Ludlow JB, Bailey LJ, et al. Accuracy of measurements of mandibular anatomy and prediction of asymmetry in panoramic radiographic images. Dentomaxillofac Radiol 2005;34(6):343–9.
12. Modgil R, Arora KS, Sharma A, et al. TMJ Arthritis Imaging: Conventional Radiograph vs. CT Scan - Is CT Actually Needed? Curr Rheumatol Rev 2019;15(2):135–40.
13. Zeng DL, Liu Y, Zhang ZG, et al. [Application of arthrography with cone-beam CT imaging in the diagnosis of temporomandibular disorders]. Zhonghua Kou Qiang Yi Xue Za Zhi 2020;55(9):634–8. Chinese.
14. Mallya SM, Lam EWN. White and pharoah's oral radiology: principles and interpretation. 8th edition. St. Louis, MO: Elsevier; 2018.
15. Barkhordarian A, Demerjian G, Chiappelli F. Translational research of temporomandibular joint pathology: a preliminary biomarker and fMRI study. J Transl Med 2020;18(1):22.
16. Bag AK, Gaddikeri S, Singhal A, et al. Imaging of the temporomandibular joint: An update. World J Radiol 2014;6(8):567–82.
17. Petscavage-Thomas JM, Walker EA. Unlocking the jaw: advanced imaging of the temporomandibular joint. AJR Am J Roentgenol 2014;203(5):1047–58.
18. Lee YH, Hong IK, Chun YH. Prediction of painful temporomandibular joint osteoarthritis in juvenile patients using bone scintigraphy. Clin Exp Dent Res 2019;5(3):225–35.
19. Hess S, Høilund-carlsen PF, Alavi A. Historic images in nuclear medicine: 1976: the first issue of clinical nuclear medicine and the first human FDG study. Clin Nucl Med 2014;39(8):701–3.

Biomechanics and Derangements of the Temporomandibular Joint

Sowmya Ananthan, BDS, DMD, MSD[a],*, Richard A. Pertes, DDS[a],
Steven D. Bender, DDS[b]

KEYWORDS

- Temporo-mandibular joint • Internal derangements • Disc displacements
- Limited mouth opening

KEY POINTS

- In disc displacement with reduction, there is an opening click (disc reduction) and a closing click (discdisplacement).
- In disc displacement with reduction with intermittent locking, there is a high probability of progression to a discdisplacement without reduction.
- In disc displacement without reduction, there is no click. The jaw is locked, with limited mandibular opening, protrusion, and lateral excursion to the contra-lateral side.

INTRODUCTION

The human temporomandibular joint (TMJ), described as a ginglymoarthrodial joint, is a highly complex synovial joint in which the two condyles function at the same time. The complex is capable of both ginglymoid and arthrodial movements. It is the only joint structure in the body with two distinct compartments separated by a fibrocartilagenous disc. The two compartments of the joint are filled with synovial fluid which provides lubrication and nutrition to the joint structures. The gliding movements, also referred to as translatory movements, occur in the upper joint compartment between the articular disc and glenoid fossa, whereas the hinge or rotary joint movements occur in the lower compartment between the disc and the condyle. The bony aspects of the complex are held together with ligaments. These ligaments surround the TMJ to form the joint capsule. The lateral aspect of the capsule is formed by the temporomandibular ligament. The joint capsule serves to limit the movements of the mandible. A more detailed description of the anatomy can be found in other chapters of this

[a] Department of Diagnostic Sciences, Center for Temporomandibular Disorders & Orofacial Pain, Rutgers School of Dental Medicine, 110 Bergen Street, Newark, NJ 07101, USA;
[b] Department of Oral and Maxillofacial Surgery, College of Dentistry, Texas A & M Health, 3302 Gaston Avenue, Dallas, TX 75246, USA
* Corresponding author.
E-mail address: ananths1@sdm.rutgers.edu

Dent Clin N Am 67 (2023) 243–257
https://doi.org/10.1016/j.cden.2022.11.004
0011-8532/23/© 2022 Elsevier Inc. All rights reserved.

dental.theclinics.com

edition. The movements of the mandible are mostly determined by the shape of the boney architecture, the muscles of mastication, the ligaments, and the unique pattern of occlusion for each individual.

The muscles of mastication consist of four paired muscle groups that include the masseter, temporalis, medial pterygoid, and lateral pterygoid muscles. The digastric muscles are not generally considered to be muscles of mastication but do serve an important role in the movement of the mandible. These muscle groups will work in concert with one another in positioning and movement of the mandible to accomplish important functions such as chewing, speaking, and swallowing. The lateral pterygoid muscle is thought to influence the articular disc position and movement due to the small portion of the superior aspect of this muscle that attaches to the disc. However, there is debate as to the amount of attachment and the significance this may have on the movement of the disc[1,2] (**Table 1**).

BIOMECHANICS OF THE TEMPOROMANDIBULAR JOINT

Movements of the mandible will cause both static and dynamic alterations in the TMJ by generating forces such as compressive, tensile, and shear loading on the articular surfaces.

The articular disc serves as a very fibrous and viscoelastic structure that allows force distribution and smooth movement of the joint in its normal arrangement during these processes. Most studies suggest that the normal disc position is where the posterior band is located at the 12'o clock position within the glenoid fossa in the closed mouth posture.[3] The force of the condyle will be directed toward the intermediate zone of the articular discwhich will lie against the anterior slope of the glenoid fossa. Anterior to the disc is the anterior attachment which joins the disc to the TMJ capsule. The posterior discattachment is sometimes referred to as the bilaminar zone. This highly vascularized tissue consists of two parts; the superior fibroelastic layer that attaches the disc to the posterior aspect of the glenoid fossa and the inferior fibrous layer that

Table 1 Muscles involved in mandibular movements	
	Action
Muscles Involved in Jaw Opening	
Digastrics	Rotation
Superior and inferior lateral pterygoids	Translation
Muscles involved in jaw closing	
Masseter	
Medial pterygoid	
Superior lateral pterygoid	Minimal involvement
Muscles involved in protrusion	
Superior and inferior lateral pterygoids	
Superficial masseter	Limited involvement
Medial pterygoid	Limited involvement
Muscles involved in lateral excursions	
Superior and inferior lateral pterygoids Medial pterygoid	Contra-lateral to the direction of movement
Masseter and temporalis	Ipsilateral: keep condyle braced within the articular fossa

attaches the disc to the posterior portion of the condylar neck. The upper and lower layers are separated by the intermediate layer, which contains loose connective tissue and attaches to the posterior wall of the joint capsule. The posterior attachment will elongate as the condyle translates anteriorly in the fossa and then shortens with jaw closing as the condyle repositions in the fossa. The disc is very tightly attached to the medial and lateral aspects of the condylar head by the discal ligaments. The disc is not attached to the medial and lateral aspects of the joint capsule. This arrangement appears to allow for a small amount of anterior and posterior rotation of the articular disc along the head of the condyle as the condyle moves within the fossa.

In the early mouth opening phase, condylar movement will occur in an inferior and anterior direction beneath the intermediate zone of the articular disc by approximately 6 to 9 mm, causing an elongation of the retro discal tissues.[4] Even with early opening, both rotation and translation will be observed in the TMJ. As mentioned, the rotation will occur between the condyle and the articular disc whereas the translation is simultaneously occurring between the disc and the fossa. The muscles involved in jaw opening include the digastric muscles (rotation) and the bilateral lateral pterygoid muscles (translation) involving both the superior and inferior aspects.[4,5] With later mouth opening the condylar movement will occur in an inferior and anterior direction loading a portion of the anterior band of the articular disc as it rotates posteriorly in relation to the condyle.[4] With jaw closing, condylar translation occurs in the posterior direction along with rotation as the mouth closes completely. The articular disc will rotate anteriorly with jaw closing. The masseter muscles as well as the medial pterygoid, temporalis, along with minimal activity of the superior aspect of the lateral pterygoid muscle are all involved in the closing action.[5] For a protrusive movement, bilateral and simultaneous contractions of the lateral pterygoid muscles involving both the superior and inferior aspects will occur. There is also some involvement of the superficial masseter muscle as well as potentially the medial pterygoid muscle.[5] This is mostly a translational movement with the articular disc interposed between the condyle and glenoid fossa. In a unilateral eccentric movement, the superior and inferior portions of the lateral pterygoid contralateral to the direction of movement of the mandible will contract. Also involved will be the masseter and temporalis muscles on the ipsilateral side keeping the ipsilateral condyle braced within the articular fossa. The medial pterygoid on the contralateral side of the direction of the movement may also be involved.[5] The condyle on the contralateral side of the direction of the mandibular movement will show translation within the articular fossa. In an ideal condyle to disc arrangement, the articular disc will remain interposed between the two structures with the load being placed primarily on the intermediate zone of the articular disc.

DERANGEMENTS OF THE TEMPOROMANDIBULAR JOINT

In a healthy joint, the posterior band of the articular disc ends at the apex of the condyle when the teeth are in occlusion. However, when the biomechanics of the joint is altered, the disc may be displaced creating an abnormal relationship between the disc, condyle, and the eminence that is often referred to as an internal derangement. Usually, the disc is displaced in an anterior or anteromedial direction, but medial, lateral, and even posterior displacements have been reported.

The disc is maintained in its proper relationship by tight discal ligaments and a self-seating capacity provided by thick posterior and anterior borders of the disc, which act as wedges holding it in position. Because the only physiologic movement occuring between the condyle and disc is rotation, any sliding movement between the disc and condyle is considered abnormal.

Several possible causes for disc displacements have been proposed, but trauma is the most common etiologic factor contributing to a change in biomechanics in the joint. It can take the form of macro-trauma from a sudden blow to the jaw, especially when the mouth is open. Most cases of internal derangement, however, are caused by micro-trauma involving mild, frequent, and repetitive forces on the joint over a prolonged period. A common example of microtrauma is bruxism.[6]

As a result of prolonged clenching, hard biting, or trauma with the teeth together, excessive pressure on the joint may cause the expression of the synovial fluid that lubricates the junction between the superior surface of the disc and the articular eminence. This may introduce a harmful frictional component into normal translatory movement and cause an adhesion to develop between these surfaces. When this occurs, the disc may become temporarily fixated to the eminence sometimes referred to as a "sticky disc".[7,8] With opening, the disc will lift off the condyle accompanied by a single-clicking noise, and lubrication to the joint surfaces will return leading to a resumption of normal joint function. But in the process of breaking the adhesion between the disc and eminence, the discal ligaments may become stretched. These ligaments do not have the property of elasticity and function to limit movement and when they become elongated, the stage is set for a disc displacement.[9]

If the disc is displaced, the inferior retrodiscal lamina, which limits anterior rotations of the disc on the condyle may also become elongated allowing the disc to become positioned more anteriorly on the condyle. Now, any pressure on the TMJ will cause thinning of the posterior border of the disc resulting in a loss of its self-seating capacity further encouraging displacement of the disc.

In the diagnostic criteria for temporomandibular disorders (DC/TMD) classification,[10] the most common intra-articular disorders involving a disc displacement include:

- Disc displacement with reduction
- Disc displacement with reduction with intermittent locking
- Disc displacement without reduction with limited opening
- Disc displacement without reduction without limited opening

Although disc displacements are presented as a series of progressively worsening clinical stages starting with disc displacement with reduction, studies indicate that few patients follow this progression.[11] Most patients remain in the initial stage of disc displacement with reduction *for years* and are able to adapt to their dysfunction with little or no discomfort.[12] Why this occurs is not clear, but it has been suggested that patients with a lack of posterior dental support, systemic ligament laxity, and parafunctional activity may be more susceptible.

DISC DISPLACEMENT WITH REDUCTION

The DC/TMD describes this stage as "An intracapsular biomechanical disorder characterized by displacement of the disc in an anterior position relative to the condylar head in the closed mouth position and the disc reduces on mouth opening with a return to a more normal position relative to the condyle on opening".

Clinical Signs and Symptoms

The most characteristic feature is a clicking, popping, or snapping sound detected with palpation during opening and closing. The opening click can occur at any point in the translatory cycle as the condyle traverses under the posterior border of the disc into a normal relationship with the disc. This is referred to as reduction or recapture of the disc. At or near the intercuspal position, a soft click may also be detected as the disc again becomes displaced. The dual opening and closing clicks are often referred to as reciprocal clicking with disc displacement on closing and disc reduction on opening (**Fig. 1**).

Disc displacement with reduction is also characterized by *deviation* of the mandibular midline toward the affected joint on early opening because of the displaced disc preventing condylar translation. With further opening, a clicking noise can be detected as the condyle passes under the posterior border of the disc indicating that the disc has been reduced. At that point in translation, the mandibular midline returns to normal. Mandibular vertical opening is usually relatively normal and any limitation on opening is due to secondary elevator masticatory muscle involvement, not mechanical obstruction by the disc.

For many years, the stage of disc displacement with reduction was thought to be a precursor to the stage of disc displacement without reduction. But studies show that most of the patients with disc displacement with reduction do not progress to disc displacement without reduction.[13] Further, disc displacement with reduction is not usually accompanied by pain.

But why is pain absent in most patients when the disc is displaced and the condyle able to press against the highly vascularized and well-innervated retrodiscal tissues in the posterior attachment, especially when the teeth are in contact? Most patients are able to adapt to this dysfunction because the posterior attachment has undergone fibrotic changes and is no longer innervated or vascularized.[14] These adaptive changes are often referred to as "pseudodisk formation" and allow the posterior attachment to function as an extension of the disc.[15,16] Therefore, when the condyle presses against the posterior attachment, there is no pain. In some cases, however, when pseudodisc adaptation does not occur, pain may be present as a result of inflammation in the posterior attachment or strained discal ligaments.

Diagnosis

The diagnosis of disc displacement with reduction is based on a history of any TMJ noise with jaw movement in the past 30 days or a patient report of jaw noise during the clinical exam. In addition, a clicking, popping, and/or snapping noise must be detected with palpation during at least one of three repetitions of opening and closing movements (DC/TMD). Joint sounds commonly occur in the general population. In the DC/TMD, the sensitivity (ie, ability of a test to correctly identify patients with the disease) for diagnosing disc displacement with reduction without imaging is 0.34 and the sensitivity (ie, ability of a test to correctly identify people without the disease) is 0.92. This indicates that most clinicians encounter difficulty diagnosing a disc displacement and questions the accuracy of using only palpation of the joint for this purpose.

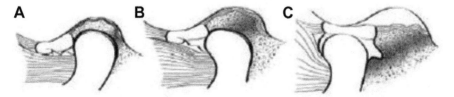

Fig. 1. Disc displacement with reduction showing late reduction of the disc in the translatory cycle. As the condyle passes under the posterior border of the disc, an opening click is usually heard. (*A*) the displaced disc in closed mouth position, (*B*) condyle passing under the posterior border of the disc. (*C*) disc reduction has been accomplished. (*From* Pertes,RA, Gross SG. Clinical Management of Temporomandibular Disorders and Orofacial Pain. Chicago, Quintessence, 1995.)

In a study involving 273 consecutive patients with TMD, clicking was detected in 143 joints using digital palpation during mouth opening and closing, but the accuracy of identifying disc displacement / with (DD/W) reduction was relatively low as verified with MRI in these patients. However, with the use of a Clicking Elimination Test the accuracy of detecting DD/W reduction significantly improved.[17] In this test, the patient to open his/her mouth until a clicking noise occurs indicating the disc has been reduced. Then the patient is instructed to close in a protruded edge-to-edge position. At that point, the disc is still reduced and when the patient opens there will be no joint noise. But if clicking is not eliminated, the patient should be asked to repeat opening and closing the mouth in a more protruded position until clicking is no longer present.

If the diagnosis is still unclear, MRI of the TMJs may be needed. To correctly diagnose DD W/red using MRI, the DC/TMD states that the posterior band of the disc should be located anterior to the 11:30 position and the intermediate zone of the disc anterior to the condylar head in maximum intercuspation. On full opening, the intermediate zone of the disc should be between the condylar head and the articular eminence (**Fig. 2**).

Management

When there is no pain and minimal interference with function, no treatment is indicated. However, it is important to educate the patient about the biomechanics involved in disc displacement and the benign nature of this disorder to allay any fears the patient might have. However, there remains a small possibility of progression to disc displacement without reduction and the patient should be periodically monitored for any changes.

Because the disc is displaced, it seemed obvious that the goal of treatment should be to restore a normal disc-condyle relationship. This led to the concept of using mandibular repositioning appliances to advance the mandible forward into a new therapeutic position to "recapture" or reduce the disc and eliminate clicking.[18] On a

Disc Displacement with Displacement
• Magnetic Resonance Imaging

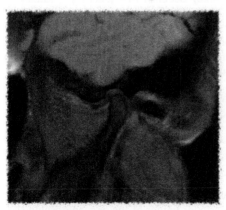 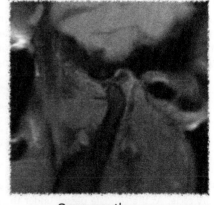

Closed mouth   Open mouth

Fig. 2. MRI showing disc displacement with reduction. Note displacement of the disc (*arrow*) anterior to the condyle in closed position and reduction of the disc to a more "normal" location between the condyle and eminence in open position.

short-term basis, mandibular repositioning appeared to be successful, but long-term efforts to permanently recapture the disc were not as successful, with studies showing that in most cases, that the disc remained displaced when the appliance was discontinued.[18,19] This result was not surprising, since a disc displacement causes irreversible elongation of the tight discal ligaments that hold the disc in place. When this is accompanied by flattening of the posterior border of the disc and a loss in shape of the disc,[20] it results in a loss of its self-seating capacity on the condyle.

Despite these limitations, anterior repositioning appliances did help to reduce pain.[21] With the mandible in a forward position, the condyle did not impinge upon the posterior attachment, thereby decreasing inflammation and pain. Not only did this relieve pressure on the posterior attachment, it also encouraged pseudodisc formation. After repositioning therapy, some clinicians advocate a second phase ("Phase II") of dental therapy to preserve the newly acquired occlusal relationship. This approach often involves extensive dental reconstruction or orthodontics and should be reserved for those few patients whose pain can only be managed by maintaining a forward mandibular position.[22] It appears that the main role of repositioning therapy may be to control pain while allowing the injured tissues to undergo adaptation.[6]

The most reasonable approach to the management of DDW/red is to concentrate on reducing pain without attempting to recapture the disc starting with a joint stabilization appliance to be worn at night. This is the most commonly used appliance for TMD and is often used for masticatory myalgia and TMJ arthralgia. However, it may also be effective for some cases of DD/W reduction as well, especially when the disc is reduced early in the translatory cycle.

This appliance is made in the patient's habitual arc of closure and is designed to provide a stable occlusal posture by creating contacts between the occlusal surface of the appliance and all opposing teeth. It does not involve any change in mandibular position. But if this approach is not effective, an anterior repositioning appliance should be fabricated mainly for use when sleeping. As pain decreases, the appliance can be gradually "walked back" and converted to a stabilization appliance. If symptoms return, repositioning therapy may need to be restarted despite the problems associated with repositioning, such as a posterior open bite.[23]

When pain is present, supportive therapy is needed. Nonsteroidal analgesic medications may be needed to reduce inflammation and if the masticatory muscles are secondarily involved, muscle relaxants can also be prescribed. The patient should be advised to follow a home regimen and decrease loading on the joint by eating softer foods, taking smaller bites, and reducing clenching of the teeth whenever possible.

CLINICS CARE POINTS

- A click on opening (disc reduction) and closing (disc displacement) is present.
- Pain is usually absent
- A relatively normal vertical opening is present
- If pain is present, management should focus on encouraging adaptive changes in the posterior attachment, not recapturing the disc

DISC DISPLACEMENT WITH INTERMITTENT LOCKING

Some patients with DD W/reduction may experience short episodes of limited mouth opening or locking. In these patients, the disc is in an anterior position relative to the condylar head when the mouth is closed, and the disc intermittently reduces with mouth opening. This stage represents a progressive deterioration of TMJ structures from the stage of DD W/reduction.

The episodes of locking occur because of additional elongation of the discal ligaments and more flattening of the posterior border of the disc. In addition, there is stretching and a loss of elasticity in the superior retro discal lamina of the posterior attachment, which is the only structure capable of retracting the disc on opening.[6]

Clinical Presentation

Joint noise is present on palpation during both opening and closing movement of the mandible. When the disc does not reduce on mouth opening, however, the jaw is locked and limited mandibular movement is present. When the jaw is locked, there will be no joint noise.

When the joint is locked and limited opening is present, the patient may have to maneuver his/her jaw to unlock the jaw and reduce the disc by moving the mandible to the contralateral side.

Diagnosis

A diagnosis of DDW/reduction with intermittent locking should be suspected when a patient reports a history of episodes of limited opening, especially upon awakening. It should be noted that these episodes may be extremely short, even momentarily. During the clinical examination, a clicking, popping or snapping noise is detected with palpation during opening and closing movements, which is indicative of DDW/red. The clicking elimination test can be used to confirm the diagnosis. Sometimes during the examination, the jaw may lock, and the clinician may have to perform a maneuver to reduce the disc. In the DC/TMD criteria for diagnosis, the sensitivity for diagnosing the disorder is 0.38 and the specificity is 0.98. However, in the authors' opinion, most cases can be diagnosed based on the history and clinical examination, and imaging is rarely needed.

Management

The prognosis is poor, with a greater likelihood of progression to disc displacement without reduction. However, some clinicians recommend the use of a maxillary appliance at night with a ramp to take pressure off the posterior attachment and encourage pseudodisc formation (**Fig. 3**).

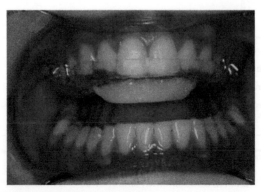

Fig. 3. Maxillary appliance with ramp.

CLINICS CARE POINTS

- Disc displacement with reduction present except when locked
- Diagnosis is mainly by the patient report of locking or if it occurs during the examination
- High probability of progression to disc displacement without opening

DISC DISPLACEMENT WITHOUT REDUCTION WITH LIMITED OPENING

In the DC/TMD, this stage is described a disorder in which the disc is in an anterior position relative to the condylar head in the closed mouth position and does not reduce on mouth opening. Medial and lateral displacement of the disc can also occur. When the disc does not reduce on opening during translation, the condyle is unable to pass under the displaced disc and there is a loss of contact between the condyle, disc, and articular eminence. Because the disc is trapped in front of the condyle, there is a limited translatory movement that is often referred to as a "closed lock." Except where acute microtrauma is involved, this stage usually represents a progressive deterioration in joint structures starting with the stage of disc displacement with reduction (**Fig. 4**).

These patients often report a history of clicking that was interrupted by periods of locking. They usually remember when the clicking stopped and limited opening and pain started. Why this progression occurs in only a small number of patients and not in most cases of disc displacement with reduction is not clear. It has been suggested that contributing factors, such as the loss of posterior dental support, systemic ligament laxity, or the presence of parafunctional habits (clenching), may play a role.

Clinical Characteristics

This stage is relatively acute and clinical examination will reveal a severely restricted opening (25–30 mm) with a marked midline *deflection* of the mandible to the side of the affected joint (ipsilateral). Protrusive excursion is also limited and accompanied by a *deflection* to the ipsilateral side (**Fig. 5**). Lateral movement to the opposite (contralateral) side is also restricted, but mandibular movement to the ipsilateral side is normal since this only requires rotational movement of the condyle and not condylar translation.

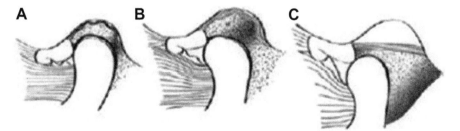

Fig. 4. Disc displacement without reduction. In the acute stage, failure to reduce the disc prevents normal condylar movement in the affected joint. With time, a more normal range of motion returns. (*A*) the displaced disc in closed mouth position. (*B*) the condyle is unable to pass under the displaced disc. (*C*) the disc is unable to reduce. (*From* Pertes, RA, Gross SG. Clinical Management of Temporomandibular Disorders and Orofacial Pain. Chicago, Quintessence, 1995.)

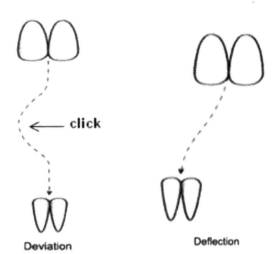

Deviation   Deflection

Fig. 5. Deviation of the incisal path is characteristic of disc displacement with reduction. The midline shifts to the ipsilateral side on opening and returns to a centered position after disc reduction. Deflection is characteristic of acute disc displacement without reduction where the midline continuously displaces to the ipsilateral side. (*From* Pertes, RA, Gross SG. Clinical Management of Temporomandibular Disorders and Orofacial Pain. Chicago, Quintessence, 1995.)

The restricted jaw movement interferes with the patient's ability to eat. Generally, this stage is accompanied by pain due to inflammation in the articular capsule, discal ligaments, and posterior attachment. Activity of the masseter and temporalis muscles on the affected side is usually increased adding to limited opening and pain.

Diagnosis

During the examination, the jaw is locked, and opening is severely limited to less than 40 mm. Because there are other causes of limited opening (hypomobility), it is important to differentiate DD W/reduction and limited opening from a masticatory elevator muscle problem. Clinically, if the elevator muscles are in spasm, only vertical opening will be limited, and lateral excursions and protrusive excursion will be normal. This contrasts with disc displacement without reduction with limited opening where vertical opening, contralateral excursion, and protrusive excursion are all restricted and only movement toward the affected joint (ipsilateral) is normal.

When opening is limited, another diagnostic test that may help in determining the nature of the restriction is the end feel. This test involves the clinician placing the thumb and middle finger between the upper and lower incisors and gently applying pressure to increase mouth opening (**Fig. 6**). If opening is increased, the end feel is considered to be *soft* and the restriction is due to masticatory muscle involvement. However, if opening is not increased, the end feel is termed *hard,* and the restricted opening is most likely due to a displaced disc that prevents condylar translation.

Management

The main goal of treatment is to decrease any pain that is present by encouraging pseudodisc formation. The chances for recapturing the disc and maintaining it on the condyle are poor because of changes in the morphology of the disc along with irreversible changes in the posterior attachment and discal ligaments. The use of an

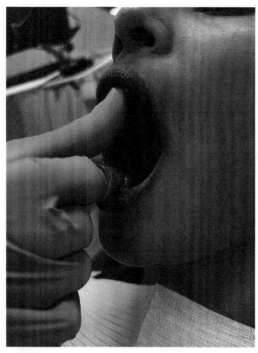

Fig. 6. Testing for end feel.

anterior repositioning appliance should be avoided because it may force the disc forward causing more pain.

Encouraging pseudodisc formation in patients with disc displacement with limited opening and leaving the disc in place is often referred to as "off the disc" treatment. It is important to note, however, that if the disc is permanently displaced, the patient is predisposed to degenerative changes in the TMJ. Without a disc between the condyle and eminence, the articular tissues covering the bony components of the joint can be distorted when subjected to heavy compressive forces. In clinical and radiological studies, a strong association was found between disc displacement without reduction and osteoarthritis.[24,25]

However, if the disc displacement was caused by a single traumatic event to a healthy joint, or occurred suddenly, an attempt should be made to reduce the disc through manual mobilization as soon as possible (see **Fig. 6**). The success of this procedure is dependent upon a functioning superior retro discal lamina, which is the only structure capable of retracting the disc.

Self-mobilization by the patient should be attempted first. The patient should be instructed to open slightly and then move the mandible as far as possible to the contralateral side. At that point, the patient should open to his/her maximum opening. If a click is heard or if the patient can open further with minimum difficulty, the disc is probably reduced. However, if after a few attempts, the disc is still displaced, manual mobilization by the clinician is indicated. With the thumb over the last molar on the side of the affected joint and the fingers placed on the inferior border of the mandible, the clinician should exert downward pressure to move the condyle inferiorly increasing the space between the condyle and eminence to allow retraction of the disc (**Fig. 7**). The patient should protrude the mandible while the clinician moves the mandible to the

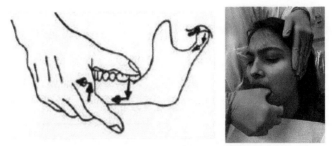

Fig. 7. Manual mobilization of the TMJ to reduce a displaced disc. Applying a downward force on the ipsilateral molars separates the condyle from the eminence to allow the superior retro discal lamina in the posterior attachment to retract the disc. Because this procedure can be painful, some patients may need a local anesthetic block of the joint.

contralateral side. If mobilization is successful, the patient should be able to achieve a normal vertical opening. At that point, cotton rolls or gauze pads should be placed between the posterior teeth on the affected side for about 10 minutes to maintain the disc reduction. As soon as possible, an appliance should be placed to move the mandible forward and allow the disc to recover its original shape. This appliance should be worn full time for about 3 to 4 days and then at night. The prognosis is fairly good, indicating that the superior retro discal lamina is still functioning and able to reduce the disc.

CLINICS CARE POINTS

- Jaw is locked causing limited mandibular opening, protrusive and lateral excursion to contralateral side
- Clicking, popping, and snapping not present in affected joint
- Usually, painful

DISC DISPLACEMENT WITHOUT REDUCTION WITHOUT LIMITED OPENING

In this stage, the disc is still displaced in an anterior position relative to the condylar head and does not reduce on opening. Although the disc is permanently displaced, as the posterior attachment elongates most patients can achieve a more normal range of motion and function normally.

Clinical Presentation

The maximum passive (operator assisted) opening is about 40 mm, which is slightly restricted. There may also be a slight deflection to the ipsilateral side and some restriction to the contralateral side.

This condition is not usually painful indicating that adaptive changes in the form of a pseudo disc occurred. A crunching or grating noise (crepitus) may be present because of degenerative changes in the joint. However, a clicking noise is absent.

Diagnosis

The patient will usually present with a prior history of jaw locking and limited mouth opening that caused difficulty with eating. Because these patients have a range of mandibular movement that is close to normal, diagnosis can be difficult, and MRI may be needed to confirm the diagnosis (**Fig. 8**). However, it is appropriate to raise

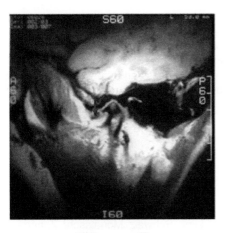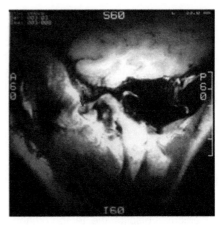

Closed   Open

Fig. 8. Disc position in anterior disc displacement without reduction, without limited open-ing, in the closed and open mouth positions. Both arrows show the anteriorly displaced disc in closed and open mouth positions in disc displacement without reduction.

the question about whether imaging is worth the expense, especially when the patient has little, if any, discomfort, and relatively normal function.

Management

Placement of a joint stabilization appliance, along with elimination of contributing fac-tors, may also help pseudodisc formation. For those patients who do not gradually achieve a normal range of opening with time, a course of physical therapy using various types of distraction procedures is recommended. This may include the use of an increasing number of tongue blades to increase the opening range, or mechan-ical devices such as the Therabite[26] or EZ-Flex. The presence of persistent pain in the joint, however, may indicate that adaptation is not occurring and an invasive proced-ure such as arthrocentesis (joint lavage) or arthroscopy should be considered.

Differential Diagnosis of Disc Displacements

Disc displacement with reduction can usually be diagnosed with considerable accu-racy by clinical examination only, without the need for imaging.[17] Most cases of disc displacement without reduction with limited opening can also be diagnosed based on clinical findings along with a prior history of clicking or recent trauma. How-ever, the accuracy of detecting disc displacement without reduction without limited opening using only history and clinical examination is not high, especially when vertical opening is close to normal and deflection to the ipsilateral side is minimal. In these cases, MRI of the TMJ may be needed to confirm the diagnosis.[27] Although a variety of electronic instruments have been developed to help evaluate disc displacements and are used by many clinicians, the validity of these diagnostic devices is questionable.

Most cases of limited mouth opening (hypomobility) are related to a masticatory muscle disorder, although a displaced disc can also limit mouth opening. From the viewpoint of a differential diagnosis, contraction of elevator muscles only restricts ver-tical opening, but does not significantly affect lateral or protrusive excursions. In contrast, an acute disc displacement (closed lock) will severely limit contralateral and protrusive movement.

Another cause of hypomobility is coronoid process hyperplasia, a rare disorder caused by progressive elongation of the coronoid process. As a result, the coronoid process is unable to pass between the zygomatic process and the lateral surface of the maxilla. Clinically, all mandibular movements will be restricted, especially protrusion.

DISCLOSURE

The authors have nothing to disclose.

REFERENCES

1. Meyenberg K, Kubik S, Palla S. Relationships of the muscles of mastication to the articular disc of the temporomandibular joint. Schweiz Monatsschr Zahnmed (1984) 1986;96(6):815–34.
2. Wilkinson TM. The relationship between the disc and the lateral pterygoid muscle in the human temporomandibular joint. J Prosthet Dent 1988;60(6):715–24.
3. Murakami S, Takahashi A, Nishiyama H, et al. Magnetic resonance evaluation of the temporomandibular joint disc position and configuration. Dentomaxillofac Radiol 1993;22(4):205–7.
4. Bhargava D, Gurjar P. Anatomy and Basic Biomechanics of the Temporomandibular Joint. In: Bhargava D, editor. Temporomandibular Joint Disorders. Singapore: Springer; 2021. p. 9–21.
5. Hargitai IA, Hawkins JM, Ehrlich AD. The Temporomandibular Joint. In: Gremillion HA, Klasse GD, editors. Temporomandibular Disorders. Berlin/Heidelberg, Germany: Springer; 2018. p. 91–107.
6. Okeson JP. Joint intracapsular disorders: diagnostic and nonsurgical management considerations. Dent Clin North Am 2007;51(1):85–103, vi.
7. Nitzan DW. The process of lubrication impairment and its involvement in temporomandibular joint disc displacement: a theoretical concept. J Oral Maxillofac Surg 2001;59(1):36–45.
8. Nitzan DW, Etsion I. Adhesive force: the underlying cause of the disc anchorage to the fossa and/or eminence in the temporomandibular joint–a new concept. J Oral Maxillofac Surg 2002;31(1):94–9.
9. Nitzan DW, Marmary Y. The "anchored disc phenomenon": a proposed etiology for sudden-onset, severe, and persistent closed lock of the temporomandibular joint. J Oral Maxillofac Surg 1997;55(8):797–802, discussion 802-3.
10. Schiffman E, Ohrbach R, Truelove E, et al. Diagnostic Criteria for Temporomandibular Disorders (DC/TMD) for Clinical and Research Applications: recommendations of the International RDC/TMD Consortium Network* and Orofacial Pain Special Interest Groupdagger. J Oral Facial Pain Headache 2014;28(1):6–27.
11. Poluha RL, Canales GT, Costa YM, et al. Temporomandibular joint disc displacement with reduction: a review of mechanisms and clinical presentation. J Appl Oral Sci 2019;27:e20180433.
12. Naeije M, Te Veldhuis AH, Te Veldhuis EC, et al. Disc displacement within the human temporomandibular joint: a systematic review of a 'noisy annoyance. J Oral Rehabil 2013;40(2):139–58.
13. Kalaykova S, Lobbezoo F, Naeije M. Two-year natural course of anterior disc displacement with reduction. J Orofac Pain Fall 2010;24(4):373–8.

14. Zhuo Z, Cai X. Results of radiological follow-up of untreated anterior disc displacement without reduction in adolescents. *Br* J Oral Maxillofac Surg 2016; 54(2):203–7.
15. Zhuo Z, Cai XY. Radiological follow-up results of untreated anterior disc displacement without reduction in adults. Int J Oral Maxillofac Surg 2016;45(3):308–12.
16. Bristela M, Schmid-Schwap M, Eder J, et al. Magnetic resonance imaging of temporomandibular joint with anterior disc dislocation without reposition - long-term results. Clin Oral Investig 2017;21(1):237–45.
17. Yatani H, Sonoyama W, Kuboki T, et al. The validity of clinical examination for diagnosing anterior disc displacement with reduction. Oral Surg Oral Med Oral Pathol Oral Radiol Endod 1998;85(6):647–53.
18. Chen HM, Liu MQ, Yap AU, et al. Physiological effects of anterior repositioning splint on temporomandibular joint disc displacement: a quantitative analysis. J Oral Rehabil 2017;44(9):664–72.
19. Lundh H, Westesson PL, Kopp S, et al. Anterior repositioning splint in the treatment of temporomandibular joints with reciprocal clicking: comparison with a flat occlusal splint and an untreated control group. Oral Surg Oral Med Oral Pathol 1985;60(2):131–6.
20. Hu YK, Yang C, Xie QY. Changes in disc status in the reducing and nonreducing anterior disc displacement of temporomandibular joint: a longitudinal retrospective study. Sci Rep 2016;6:34253.
21. Ma Z, Xie Q, Yang C, et al. Can anterior repositioning splint effectively treat temporomandibular joint disc displacement? Sci Rep 2019;9(1):534.
22. de Leeuw R, Boering G, Stegenga B, et al. TMJ articular disc position and configuration 30 years after initial diagnosis of internal derangement. J Oral Maxillofac Surg 1995;53(3):234–41, discussion 241-2.
23. Kai S, Kai H, Tabata O, et al. The significance of posterior open bite after anterior repositioning splint therapy for anteriorly displaced disc of the temporomandibular joint. Cranio 1993;11(2):146–52.
24. Kurita K, Westesson PL, Yuasa H, et al. Natural course of untreated symptomatic temporomandibular joint disc displacement without reduction. J Dent Res 1998; 77(2):361–5.
25. Dias IM, Cordeiro PC, Devito KL, et al. Evaluation of temporomandibular joint disc displacement as a risk factor for osteoarthrosis. Int J Oral Maxillofac Surg 2016; 45(3):313–7.
26. Maloney GE, Mehta N, Forgione AG, et al. Effect of a passive jaw motion device on pain and range of motion in TMD patients not responding to flat plane intraoral appliances. Cranio 2002;20(1):55–66.
27. Yatani H, Suzuki K, Kuboki T, et al. The validity of clinical examination for diagnosing anterior disc displacement without reduction. Oral Surg Oral Med Oral Pathol Oral Radiol Endod 1998;85(6):654–60.

Pathogenesis and Differential Diagnosis of Temporomandibular Joint Disorders

Junad Khan, DDS, MSD, MPH, PhD[a],*, Steven R. Singer, DDS[b],
Andrew Young, DDS, MSD[c],
Naruthorn Tanaiutchawoot, DMD, MSD[b],
Mythili Kalladka, BDS, MSD[a], Mel Mupparapu, DMD, MDS, DipABOMR[d]

KEYWORDS

- Fibromyalgia • Chronic overlapping pain conditions • Comorbid
- Temporomandibular disorder

KEY POINTS

- Temporomandibular joint disorders (TMDs) are often chronic in nature, and underlying mechanisms are poorly understood.
- TMDs can mimic as aodontogenic pain and result in unnecessary treatment and financial burden.
- TMDs can be challenging to diagnose and manage. A proper understanding and training can better help manage the patient.

INTRODUCTION

Temporomandibular disorders (TMDs) affect approximately 11.5 million individuals in the United States, entailing a significant burden on economic and health care resources. The annual incidence of clinically verified TMDs is estimated to be 4%. However, this may reflect a "symptom iceberg."[1] The condition may have a significant association with age and presents a similar incidence in men and women, with a nonsignificant higher incidence in women. The condition also has a significantly higher incidence in African Americans and whites in comparison to Asians. The variations may be explained by an incidence-prevalence bias and study design.[2] In 1992, the Research Diagnostic

[a] Orofacial Pain and TMJD, Eastman Institute for Oral Health, 625 Elmwood Avenue, Rochester, NY 14620, USA; [b] Department of Diagnostic Sciences Division of Oral & Maxillofacial Radiology, Rutgers School of Dental Medicine, 110 Bergen Street | PO Box 1709, Newark, NJ 07101-1709, USA; [c] Arthur A. Dugoni School of Dentistry, University of the Pacific, San Francisco, CA, USA; [d] Penn Dental Medicine, 240 S 40th Street, Philadelphia, PA 19104, USA
* Corresponding author.
E-mail address: Junad_khan@urmc.rochester.edu

Dent Clin N Am 67 (2023) 259–280
https://doi.org/10.1016/j.cden.2022.10.001
0011-8532/23/© 2022 Elsevier Inc. All rights reserved.

Criteria for Temporomandibular Disorders (RDC/TMD) was developed. RDC/TMD categorized TMDs into Axis I and Axis II. Axis I described the common physical TMD signs and symptoms, whereas Axis II includes conditions that relate to the psychosocial and behavior disorders. In 2008 to 2011, RDC/TMD was assessed and validated. Although Axis II seemed to be reliable and valid, Axis I was redeveloped to be a validated diagnostic criterion for clinicians and researchers and is now known as the Diagnostic Criteria for Temporomandibular Disorders (DC/TMD).[3,4]

The etiopathogenesis of TMDs is complex and involves an interplay of multiple factors across various biological, psychological, social, and environmental domains in the backdrop of genetic influences. The multiple factors may exert their influence over time, resulting in manifestation, progression, remission, or exacerbations of the condition.[1,5] Early theories were mechanistic and focused on the role of mechanistic occlusal factors as the primary factor in the genesis of these conditions. Current scientific evidence has refuted and shown a very small to no role of occlusion in the genesis of TMDs and resulted in the shift of theories from biomechanistic models toward biopsychosocial models.[6–8] The role of peripheral and central nociceptive inputs; environmental, genetic factors; and interplay of biopsychosocial risk factors in the initiation, sustenance, and progression of these conditions is currently hypothesized to play a major role in evolution of TMDs.[1]

In spite of having validated diagnostic guidelines, insights into various pathophysiological mechanisms and proper management of TMDs are still elusive and controversial. This information is crucial for successful pain management and to prevent the new incidence or recurrences in new or existing patients with TMD. The objective of the present article is to provide a comprehensive evidence-based literature review on the proposed pathophysiological mechanisms implicated in the genesis of TMDs and the clinical implications of the same following the classification guidelines as per the DC/TMD.

CAUSE AND RISK FACTORS

The Orofacial Pain: Prospective Evaluation and Risk Assessment (OPPERA) study was one of the most comprehensive studies to date assessing risk factors using prospective cohort, case-control, and nested case-control study designs. OPPERA studies enabled significant inferences on risk factors and associations playing a vital role in the initiation and sustenance of TMDs. The prospective cohort study explored the temporal sequence of risk factors and onset of TMDs, whereas the case-control study design provided information on significant associations between risk factors and TMD. Comorbid health conditions, somatic symptoms, and nonpainful orofacial symptoms emerged as the strongest predictors for incident TMDs.[9–11]

Comorbid health conditions included a list of approximately 20 different health conditions administered as a screening questionnaire, and ill-defined, painful or nonpainful conditions and cigarette smoking emerged as additional risk factors for TMDs.[12] Hormonal contraceptive initiation also increased the risk of development of subsequent TMDs, headaches, and craniofacial pain, which reduced on cessation.[13]

Self-reports by patients were stronger predictors than examiner assessments. Self-reports of temporomandibular joint (TMJ) noises and multiple parafunctional habits as assessed by the Oral Behavioral Checklist were very strong indicators of chronic TMDs and incident TMDs.[14] Multiple parafunctional habits may result in a threshold effect, elevating the risk of patients for TMDs possibly through mechanisms including central dysregulation, reduction in proprioception and motor inhibition, enhanced motor activation, and constant psychophysiological reactivity.[15] The extrinsic or intrinsic injury also increased the odds of developing TMDs significantly, and single trauma had a higher impact compared with multiple injuries to the jaw.[16] The nested case-control study reported that pressure pain thresholds were not reliable indicators of incident TMD, rather coincided with onset and progression.[17]

Sleep quality was a significant factor for incident TMD. The rate of incident TMD increased 40% for every standard deviation reduction in quality of sleep.[12] Patients with first-onset TMD had preceding OSA symptoms and 73% higher hazards of developing TMDs.[18] Poor sleep quality has been hypothesized to increase the perception of stress and additionally has a significant direct impact on pain perception through its effect on immune, metabolic, and inflammatory pathways.[19] Somatic and global psychological symptoms were the most robust psychological risk predictors for incident TMD. Previous life events, levels of perceived and measured stress, and negative effects also had important implications.[20] Previous studies have also shown that health anxiety in adults and life satisfaction, somatization, and depression in adolescents may play a role in the development of chronic orofacial pain.[21–23] Somatic symptoms also exhibited strong associations with several chronic overlapping pain conditions (COPC) and individual COPC,[24] although the exact mechanism and role of somatic symptoms in the evolution of TMD are under scrutiny. Somatic symptoms may also alter biological pathways through their effects on the inflammatory and immune pathways, and certain risk factors such as parafunctional habits may induce somatic symptoms or somatic symptoms may be manifestations of physiologic perturbations and these may act in cohort with other risk factors and play a role in initiation and sustenance or contribute to the chronicity of TMDs.[15,25,26] Patients with new-onset TMD may also exhibit greater pain and symptoms and exhibit deteriorating psychological parameters, whereas patients with chronic TMD may exhibit better biopsychosocial parameters signifying engagement of coping and adaptation skills, suggesting evolution of biopsychosocial parameters as the condition evolves, persists, or resolves.[27] The transition from acute to chronic TMDs may also be facilitated by processes such as catastrophizing.

Genes are upstream determinants of biological intermediate phenotypes that may act with environmental factors and produce downstream phenotypic effects, increasing an individual's predisposition to TMDs.[5] Studies have reported that single-nucleotide polymorphisms (SNPs) affecting the serotonergic pathway and gene-environment interaction on stress and pain were modified by the catechol O-methyltransferase (COMT). SNPs in the glucocorticoid receptor gene and serotonin receptor gene have been implicated through their action on the hypothalamic-pituitary-adrenal axis and affective, nociceptive pathways, respectively. The OPPERA study also implicated four other novel and previously unreported SNPs as risk factors for TMDs; this included voltage-gated sodium channel Nav1.1 alpha subunit, angiotensin-I–converting enzyme, prostaglandin-endoperoxide synthase 1 gene, and amyloid beta (A4) precursor protein.[28] However, it has been suggested that the complexity of TMDs may involve multiple SNPs acting through distinct biological pathways. For instance, it has been suggested that in localized TMD, the genetic interactions may activate peripheral serotonergic pathways causing local hyperalgesia but with significant counteraction by the central serotonergic pathways limiting widespread effects seen in TMDs with additional widespread body pain on palpation. Genetic factors may also play a role in modulating inflammatory responses, nociceptive sensitivity, and psychological and autonomic responses.

TMDs are no longer considered a localized condition. It may have a strong association with certain chronic overlapping pain syndromes such as fibromyalgia (FM), and the association may be influenced by the number of chronic overlapping pain conditions. In patients developing incident TMD, headache frequency and prevalence, specifically migraine, increased.[29] The overlap between COPCs was more significant for musculoskeletal conditions such as TMDs, low back pain, and FM. In addition to the overlap of pain conditions in the body and orofacial pain, a significantly higher anatomic overlap has been reported, especially in craniocervical pain reflecting differential amplification of pain inputs based on anatomic locations.[30] Segmental central sensitization (somatosensory inputs to the central nervous system (CNS) are segmentally organized and thus sensitization may alter across the neuroaxis, resulting in pain symptoms in specific sites) has also been suggested as a possible mechanism in several pain conditions with anatomic overlap.[31] Convergence of afferent nociceptive inputs at the level of the cervical first dorsal horn has been suggested as a plausible segmental sensitization mechanism in craniocervical pain conditions such as TMDs, headache, neck pain, and whiplash injuries.[32] In addition, cortical reorganization due to continued nociceptive inputs and activation of afferent pain pathways may play a role in pain processing and also contribute to this phenomenon.[30,33,34]

Significant lines of evidence seem to point to the role of peripheral and central sensitization in the evolution of painful TMDs. Painful TMDs may be one of the pathways contributing to increased synaptic efficacy of nociceptive neurons and thus drive upregulation of pathways contributing to central sensitization.[1] Inflammatory mediators including serotonin, prostaglandin E2, bradykinin, and histamine seem to show involvement in pain development in patients with muscle pain. Some studies showed the elevation of tumor necrosis factor alpha (TNF-α), interleukin-1 (IL-1), and IL-6 levels in synovial fluid of patients with TMD pain.[35,36] Upregulation of proinflammatory cytokines such as TNF-α, interleukin- IL-6, 1β (IL-1β), and monocyte chemoattractant protein-1 may activate nociceptors and this coupled with downregulation of anti-inflammatory cytokines and omentin has been suggested to play a role in the development of pain.[37–43] In addition, some nociceptive neuropeptides such as substance P, calcitonin gene–related peptide (CGRP), neuropeptide Y, and vasoactive intestinal peptide have also been shown to correlate with TMJ degeneration if imbalanced. Free radical such as reactive oxygen species also plays an important role in TMJ disease.[44]

Pain amplification that may occur as a consequence of enhanced pain facilitatory pathways in the peripheral/central nervous system or impaired modulatory pathways has also been implicated.[45] Pain amplification may be determined by genotypic or phenotypic interaction with the environment and risk factors. Acute TMDs may thus involve peripheral sensitization through injury or oral parafunctional behavior with subsequent activation of nociceptors in the masticatory tissues or it may involve dysregulation of systems beyond the local site with a more central mechanism. Peripheral mechanisms may have a more significant role in the initiation of localized TMDs, whereas the involvement of central mechanisms (central sensitization, neuroplasticity, cortical reorganization) may contribute to the persistence and chronicity of TMDs marked with widespread symptoms. Central sensitization and downregulation of modulatory pathways has also been proposed to play an important role.[15,46,47] Cluster analysis in the case-control OPPERA group has identified 3 different clusters: adaptive, pain sensitive (characterized by greater experimental pain sensitivity), and global clusters (characterized by heightened psychological distress and pain sensitivity) of patients with TMD. Analysis of the TMD cases and controls revealed that an overwhelming majority of TMD cases encompassed global symptoms and pain-sensitive clusters (91.5%), whereas a significant proportion of controls (41.2%) could be classified into the adaptive cluster. The global symptom cluster had a greater predilection for developing first-onset TMD, and the global symptom and pain-sensitive cluster exhibited grater, functional limitation, increased pain, and multiple comorbidities.[48]

A proper diagnosis of TMDs is considered the first important step to allow re-searchers to develop well-designed rigorous studies with reliable and validated infer-ences, which can then be applied by clinicians to enable evidence-based management of TMDs. At present, the standard diagnostic guideline recommended for clinicians and researchers is the DC/TMD. This section will only describe Axis I of the classification of TMDs. As per DC/TMD protocol, TMDs can be categorized into 2 dual axes. Accordingly, as per Axis I protocol, TMDs can be categorized into four major categories including temporomandibular joint disorders, masticatory mus-cle disorders, headaches, and associated structures. In this article, the authors pro-vide an overview of the pathophysiologic mechanisms as per Axis 1 DC/TMD[49] (**Figs. 1** and **2**).

JOINT PAIN
Arthralgia

The diagnosis of pain in the TMJ is termed "arthralgia." It could be confirmed by the repro-duction of chief complaint with TMJ palpation and/or with jaw movement. The palpation force recommended by DC/TMD during TMJ examination should be around 1 kg/cm^2. It is described as joint pain affected by functional or parafunctional jaw movements.

Arthritis

Arthritis is a localized joint pain condition presenting with characteristics of inflamma-tion or infection. In addition to pain, if the clinical presentation shows signs of inflam-mation including redness, swelling, or increased skin temperature, the diagnosis "arthritis" shall be made instead. It is often secondary to mechanical, metabolic, infec-tious, and/or inflammatory factors.[50]

JOINT DISORDERS
Degenerative Joint Disease, Disc Displacements, and Subluxation

The diagnostic criteria for the degenerative joint disease do not include pain; the diag-nosis refers to the TMJ's erosion of the articular surface. If pain is present, this is

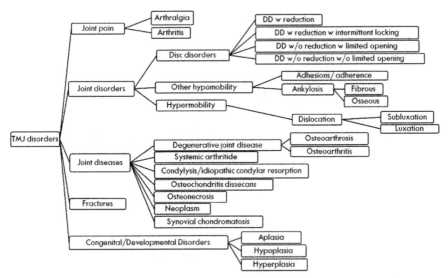

Fig. 1. The flow chart shows the classification of temporomandibular joint disorders.

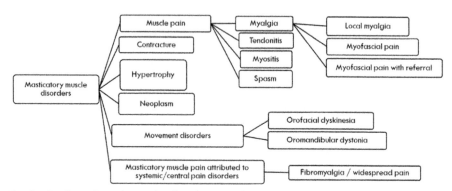

Fig. 2. The flow chart shows the classification of masticatory muscle disorders.

referred to as "temporomandibular joint pain attributed to degenerative joint disease" in the ICOP[1]; in the DC/TMD, for this presentation, two diagnoses would be given: "degenerative joint disease" and "arthralgia.[3]"

The same diagnostic criteria approach holds for pain with TMJ disc displacement and subluxation: if they are painful, the diagnoses "TMJ pain" or "arthralgia" are attached. TMJ subluxation and disc displacement with reduction (DDWR) have very similar presentations. Subluxation has a loud, late pop with a wide opening and may have a closing pop as well. DDWR can have a loud pop, or a fainter click, and these noises may occur anywhere from early to late in the condylar translation.[3] One distinguishing factor is the intensity of the joint sound. Only DDWR can have a faint click; a louder pop can be either. Another distinguishing feature is the timing of the pop. An early pop is not a feature of subluxation, so would have to be diagnosed as DDWR; a late pop can be either. Lastly, the direction of jaw deviation can help differentiate. In subluxation, the mandible deviates toward the side contralateral to the pop, at the time of the pop; in DDWR, the mandible deviates toward the side ipsilateral to the pop.

If the disc is displaced anterior to the condylar head in a closed mouth position and is recaptured to the normal position while opening, then this condition should be diagnosed as anterior DDWR. In instances when the disc is displaced anteriorly to the condylar head in mouth closing position and maintained anteriorly even with mouth opening, this condition should be diagnosed as "anterior disc displacement without reduction." Several hypotheses have been proposed, and one of the hypotheses on etiopathogenesis in articular disc disorders suggests that it may involve alterations in the intraarticular lubrication, leading to increased articular friction. However, this may become symptomatic generally only in a predisposed joint with other risk factors (trauma, alterations in joint or disc morphology, dynamics, hypermobility, and so forth). Trauma may induce an inflammatory response primarily in the retro discal tissue and damage the ligaments and posterior attachment of the joint, enhancing susceptibility to articular disc disorders. Instances of articular overloading exceeding the adaptive remodeling capacity of the joint may also induce changes in the articular disc that has limited remodeling capacity in comparison to the bony structures of the joint and lead to articular disc disorders.[51]

Temporomandibular Joint Hypomobility

TMJ hypomobility is a condition that does not allow the jaw to be able to move to the normal limit, may be a sequela of intraarticular fibrotic adhesions or due to fibrous or bony ankylosis. In most instances, they may be sequelae of trauma (macrotrauma/

fractures) and occasionally due to systemic diseases (such as psoriatic or rheumatoid arthritis, fibrodysplasia ossificans progressiva,[52–54] infections [middle ear and mastoid]).[55,56]

Temporomandibular Joint Hypermobility

It is a condition characterized by the ability of the jaw to move beyond the normal limit (hypermobility). Pathophysiologic alterations in the supporting structures (ligaments, bony, and muscle components) of TMJ have been proposed to be the primary factors in the etiopathogenesis of hypermobility disorders; this may be secondary to trauma, systemic conditions, and other factors.[57] Animal models of traumatic TMJ hypermobility have demonstrated changes in the synovium of the upper joint compartment, deposition of fibrin in inflamed synovial tissues, adhesions, capillary hyperemia, the proliferation of surface cells, and synovitis.[58] A systematic review on the role of generalized joint hypermobility (GJH) in TMD is still unclear and suggests that the condition warrants further research.[59] GJH may be seen in conditions such as Ehlers Danlos syndrome. GJH may be associated with several conditions affecting the locomotor system such as myalgia, arthralgia, soft tissue lesions, dislocations, traumatic synovitis, and so forth. It has been proposed that the increased range of movement may overload the joint and increase susceptibility to mechanical damage, or the alterations in the quality of collagen in these disorders may terminate in degenerative changes or clinical manifestations of the condition. GJH may frequently be associated with TMDs such as osteoarthritis.

JOINT DISEASES

Imaging of the TMJ is an important aspect of diagnosis especially if the bony components of the joint are affected. Plain digital radiography (planar radiography), cone-beam computed tomography (CBCT), multidetector computed tomography, and MR imaging can be used to image joints, and functional imaging such as PET and PET-CT imaging can be used to identify malignant disorders. Three-dimensional reconstructions help in displaying the TMJ in all 3 dimensions (**Fig. 3**).

Osteoarthrosis and Osteoarthritis

These are degenerative joint conditions. According to DC/TMD, both conditions show similar signs of TMJ degeneration, but osteoarthrosis presents without arthralgia, whereas osteoarthritis presents with arthralgia. Often the terms are used interchangeably. Osteoarthritis is a multifactorial condition with a complex pathogenesis involving sustained inflammation. Mechanical and metabolic factors may initiate early damage of articular cartilage, triggering immune and biochemical responses in the hard and soft tissues of the joint. Immune cells may release inflammatory mediators including cytokines and chemokines and activate the complement system, causing the release of factors that can damage articular cartilage including prostaglandin E and matrix metalloproteinase. The local inflammatory response can damage and degrade the articular cartilage and cause remodeling changes in the subchondral bone[60] (**Figs. 4 and 5**).

Systemic Arthritides

Systemic arthritides are pain and structural changes secondary to joint inflammation resulting from systemic conditions such as juvenile idiopathic arthritis, rheumatoid arthritis spondyloarthropathies (psoriatic arthritis, ankylosing spondylitis, Reiter

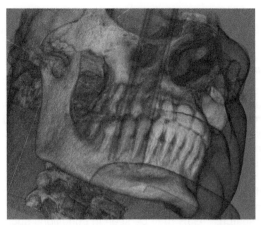

Fig. 3. Three-dimensional reconstruction (Recon) of the right TMJ using CBCT.

syndrome, infectious arthritis), and crystal-induced (chondrocalcinosis, gout) and autoimmune conditions (lupus erythematosus, Sjögren syndrome, scleroderma).[61]

TMJ arthritis caused by systemic disease is generally painful, and diagnosis is made by a combination of clinical presentation, consideration for existing systemic disease, imaging, and serologic studies.[61,62]

In cases where the joints are completely degenerated or destroyed, a total joint replacement is recommended, which will bring back function and reduce pain in the patient (**Fig. 6**).

Idiopathic Condylar Resorption

The etiopathogenesis is still unclear, and it has been suggested to be idiopathic (**Figs. 7–10**). Previously, estrogen, reduced 17β-estradiol levels, mechanical loading, and dysfunctional remodeling of the condyle have been suggested as possible factors. Condylar resorption may also be secondary to surgeries such as orthognathic surgery and often these cases are also classified into the category of ICR. A systematic review reported that at present there is a lack of evidence to suggest estrogen deficiency as a contributor. However, the quality of evidence is low and the investigators suggest further rigorous studies to investigate the matter.[63]

Osteochondritis Dissecans

Osteochondritis dissecans is the presence of loose osteochondral fragments in the joint due to detachment of cartilage and a fragment of bone from a bony extremity. The pathophysiological mechanisms are yet to be elucidated in the TMJ.[61]

Osteonecrosis

This condition is characterized by necrotic bone and pain. When it occurs in the TMJ condyle, it is difficult to distinguish from arthritis. When it occurs in nonarticular areas of the maxillofacial region, where arthritis does not occur, and where it can be clinically observed when it penetrates the soft tissue, it is more easily diagnosed. The history generally must be positive for trauma or surgery and antiresorptive medication or radiation.[61]

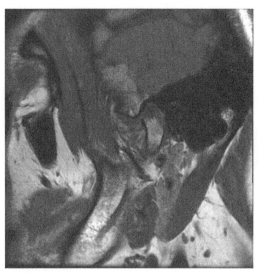

Fig. 4. T1W sagittal MR image showing significant erosion and osteophyte formation in the superior and anterior aspects of the condylar head due to degenerative joint disease.

BENIGN BONE TUMORS

Although often asymptomatic, these conditions may present with swelling when painful. Osteoid osteoma may be confused with myofascial orofacial pain (MOP). It progressively worsens, is often worst at night, and is relieved by nonsteroidal antiinflammatory drugs (NSAIDs). However, pain intensity is unrelated to activity, which may cue the diagnostician to a non-TMD diagnosis.[62] Osteoblastoma has continuous pain that is not relieved by NSAIDs. Clinically aggressive bone lesions

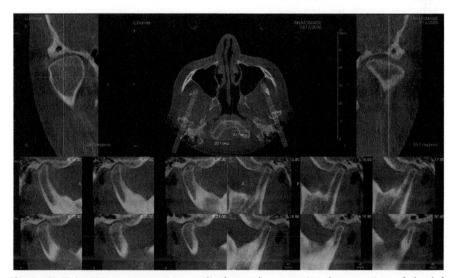

Fig. 5. CBCT in TMJ reconstruction mode shows the extensive degeneration of the left condyle in comparison to the normal right condyle.

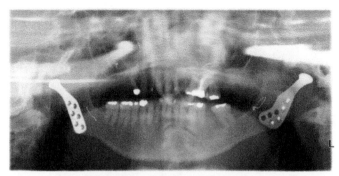

Fig. 6. A panoramic radiograph showing total joint replacement of the TMJ bilaterally in a patient with significant TMJ arthritis, leading to the destruction of left and right condyles.

such as ameloblastomas (**Fig. 11**) can essentially affect the body or the ramus of the mandible and can mimic orofacial pain due to bone expansion and compression of the neurovascular bundles.

Synovial Chondromatosis

In synovial enchondromatosis, metaplasia of the TMJ synovial tissue results in cartilaginous nodules that may detach, becoming loose bodies. In osteochondromatosis, the nodules are calcified. Pain, TMJ swelling, progressive limitation in mouth opening, posterior open bite, and/or crepitus may develop. Although clinically it can be confused with simple TMJ pain, or with lateral pterygoid spasm, differentiation is achieved by imaging.[61]

The pathogenesis involves chronic inflammation and metaplasia of the synovial membrane progressing to a stage of synovial progressive metaplasia with detached particles (active chondrocytes partially encased in the synovial membrane), and finally, only detached particles are present.[64] Synovial macrophages, tenascin, transforming

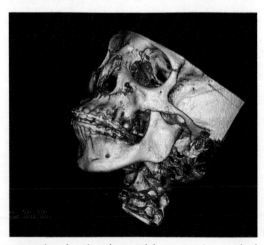

Fig. 7. CBCT 3D reconstruction showing the condylar resorption on the left. The patient had bilateral condylar resorption.

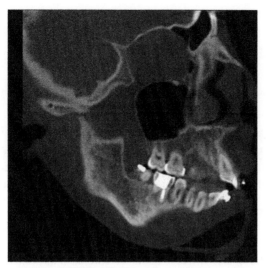

Fig. 8. Right oblique sagittal CBCT slice showing the condylar resorption on the right side.

growth factor beta, and fibroblastic growth factor receptor have also been implicated in the etiopathogenesis of SC due to their role in chondrogenesis.[65–67]

MALIGNANT BONE TUMORS

Osteosarcoma can occur in jaw bones, although such occurrences are rare; the pain often begins after an injury and may fluctuate over weeks to months. Langerhans cell histiocytosis may have a soft tissue mass and pain. Multiple myeloma presents with osteolytic lesions and bone pain.[62]

Primary malignant lesions or metastatic lesions can be detected via nuclear medicine–based scans, more precisely via PET-CT, and **Fig. 12** shows the active uptake of radiolabeled glucose absorption at the potentially malignant site near the right ramus.

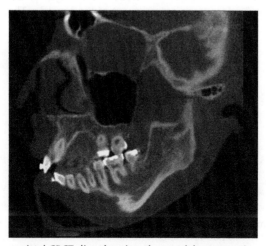

Fig. 9. Left oblique sagittal CBCT slice showing the condylar resorption on the left side.

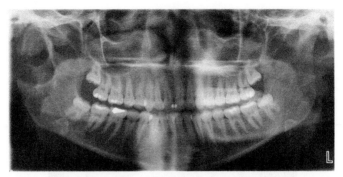

Fig. 10. A variant of idiopathic condylar resorption—this resorptive process included part of the right ramus, condylar neck, and the head of the condyle. The patient only had mild discomfort during the opening and closing of the mouth.

SINUSITIS

Inflammation in the sinus, whether acute or chronic (**Fig. 13**), is typically painful. Although the maxillary sinuses are not immediately adjacent to the masticatory muscles, sinusitis-related pain can be confused with masseter, medial pterygoid, or lateral pterygoid MOP if the pain is diffuse enough or if it refers to the proximity of those muscles. Sinusitis pain differs from MOP in that it is not altered with jaw function or palpation, does not limit the range of motion, often worsens with bending forward, and usually has a history of current or recent allergies or upper respiratory tract infection.[68,69]

Fractures: if the patients report a history of traumatic incidence, fractures of jaw-related structures should be considered. The diagnosis should be proposed with radiographic evidence of fracture. On occasion, the fractured portion of the elongated styloid process can also lead to diffuse pain in the neck and may radiate to the ipsilateral TMJ. The reliable and valid radiographs suggested in DC/TMD to confirm the fracture are CT scan or CBCT imaging.

Congenital: anatomic abnormality of the TMJ condyle may be encountered. In the case of a total absence of the condyle, either ipsilateral or bilaterally, the diagnosis should be "aplasia." "Hypoplasia" describes the condyle to be smaller, whereas normal "hyperplasia" refers to an enlargement of the condyle. These conditions can

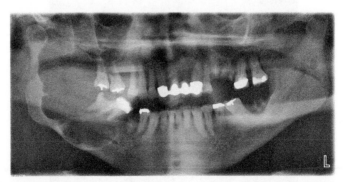

Fig. 11. A panoramic radiograph shows significant destruction of the right body of the mandible and right ramus due to ameloblastoma. A small well-defined radiolucency within the left ramus is the medial sigmoid depression, which is developmental.

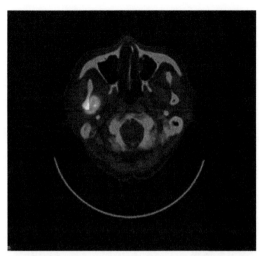

Fig. 12. An FDG PET-CT image of a metastatic tumor near the right ramus closer to the condyle showing a high amount of uptake of the radionuclide tracer. FDG, fluorodeoxyglucose.

affect unilateral or bilateral TMJs. Congenital TMDs may be isolated occurrences (intrauterine defects during the prenatal period of TMJ development) or part of various syndromes affecting first and second branchial arches such as Treacher Collins syndrome, Goldenhar syndrome, Hallermann-Streiff syndrome, Hemifacial microsomia, Hurler syndrome, Morquio syndrome, Proteus syndrome, and Auriculocondylar syndrome.[67] Condylar hyperplasia is secondary to a nonneoplastic proliferative increase in normal cells, resulting in overdevelopment of condyle or entire mandible/facial bones.[61]

MASTICATORY MUSCLE DISORDERS

According to DC/TMD, myofascial pain is a subcategory under the diagnosis of myalgia. Myalgia can be diagnosed based on the patient's chief complaint of pain in the masticatory muscle location, and the pain can be reproduced by muscle palpation. Recommended force for muscle palpation suggested in DC/TMD is 1 kg/cm^2. If the pain seems to be localized under the palpation area, the diagnosis of "local myalgia" should be given. If the pain spreads beyond the palpation area but is restricted to the muscle boundary, it is recognized as "myofascial pain without referral." In the case that the pain travels beyond the boundary of palpated muscle and refers to a remote area, which is perceived and reported by the patients, the diagnosis should be "myofascial pain with referral."

Myofascial Pain

Pain with jaw function (whether the force of chewing or the act of stretching the jaw), pain with palpation, and limitation in jaw range of motion due to pain distinguish masticatory MOP from headaches and neuropathic pain, which at times overlap with MOP by location and pain quality.[62] Neuropathic pain can also be triggered by jaw function or palpation but tend to be disproportional to the stimulus. Trigeminal neuralgia, for example, is often characterized by explosive pain with normally innocuous touch or gentle jaw movements.[62] MOP pain, on the other hand, increases in proportion to

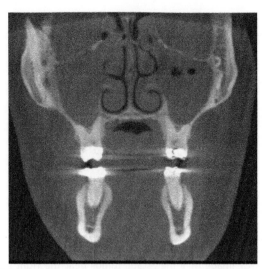

Fig. 13. Coronal CBCT at the level of the maxillary sinuses showing severe bilateral maxillary sinusitis.

the degree or duration of force applied during chewing, the distance of jaw movement, or the amount of pressure applied during palpation. Some muscles, such as the medial and lateral pterygoid muscles, are difficult or impossible to palpate; these muscles therefore can only be tested with load or range-of-motion testing.[61]

Myalgia

Although specific pathophysiologic mechanisms for masticatory myalgia in the orofacial region are yet to be completely elucidated, they may share certain common mechanisms involved in myofascial pain. It is currently hypothesized that myofascial pain is initiated and sustained by the presence of myofascial trigger points that are hyperirritable spots in taut bands of muscle and occur when the adaptive capacity of muscles is exceeded by functional demands. Excess acetylcholine, CGRP-related mechanism, and acidic environment may lead to dysfunctional neuromuscular endplates and result in sustained sarcomere contraction; this may lead to restriction in blood flow, local hypoxia, the cumulation of waste products, and a deficit of adenosine triphosphate; this causes an energy crisis and the formation of trigger points. Various other mechanisms and theories have been proposed including the role of peripheral and central sensitization, Cinderella theory (hierarchical recruitment patterns of muscle fibers result in smallest fibers being subjected to longest duration of contraction and increased susceptibility to initiating energy crisis in phasic muscles), and shift theory (tonic muscles with the shift pattern of recruitment are susceptible with prolonged periods of contraction and insufficient relaxation), the possible role of descending modulation.[70]

Myositis

Muscle pain associated with signs of inflammation is referred to as myositis. It is generally secondary to trauma, infection, or in chronic cases, it may be secondary autoimmune conditions. The allogenic inflammatory mediators released at the site of inflammation/tissue damage can lower the detection threshold and result in peripheral sensitization and pain as mentioned in the introductory section. This infectious and/or inflammatory muscle condition is usually caused by direct trauma or acute infection to the muscle or a chronic autoimmune disease. It must be accompanied by edema, erythema, or increased temperature of the muscle. Serologic testing may be done, which may reveal elevated inflammatory markers such as creatine kinase.[61]

Tendonitis

It is described as pain restricted to the masticatory tendon, most commonly temporal tendon with replication of pain with functional or parafunctional movements of the jaw.[61] The pain of this inflammatory condition seems as MOP, differing only by the precise location of the pain. Differentiation relies on a strong familiarity with the anatomy of masticatory muscles and associated structures. Due to varied anatomy amongst individuals, location of the muscle-tendon junction, tendonitis and MOP cannot always be distinguished with absolute certainty. The temporalis tendon is the most common site of tendonitis in the masticatory system.[61]

Spasms

Spasm is defined by the DC/TMD as a "sudden, involuntary, reversible tonic contraction of a muscle." It must be accompanied by pain and limitation of the jaw opening (<40 mm) and/or laterotrusion (<7 mm), which differentiates it from MOP; if a patient has muscle pain without a limitation in jaw range, the diagnosis is simply MOP.[61] TMJ pain attributed to a disc displacement without reduction can also cause limitation in jaw range, but spasm differs in that the sense of pain and range limitation is felt within a muscle and the offending event occurred in the muscle. If those parameters are too unclear for a definitive diagnosis of spasm over a disc displacement, the description of "TMJ pain" discussed in this article may be used to further differentiate.[62]

Temporomandibular Joint Pain

TMJ pain (also known as "arthralgia" in the DC/TMD), similar to MOP, is characterized by pain with jaw function, pain with palpation, and limitation in jaw range of motion due to pain. When the pain is located in a site remote from the TMJ, differentiation is relatively simple. However, MOP can occur in the proximity of the TMJ, as portions of every masticatory muscle pass near the TMJ. In such cases, other parameters of differentiation are needed. If palpation of the TMJ causes pain, TMJ pain is confirmed[61,62]; if palpation of the TMJ does not cause pain, that does not definitively rule out TMJ pain, as most of the TMJ cannot be reached for palpation. TMJ arthralgia is more likely to be aggravated by jaw laterotrusion, so that test can suggest TMJ arthralgia rather than MOP. If a pop or click is present and hurts, or if the patient reports the pain to be in the same location as the joint sounds, TMJ pain is very likely.

Contracture

Extended immobilization periods following surgery, trauma, radiation therapy, or infection may result in fibrosis of muscle fibers or supporting structures such as tendons and ligaments, resulting in painless limitation unless the involved muscle is extended beyond the functional length.[61] This shortening of a muscle due to fibrosis of the muscle, ligaments, or tendons may seem similar to MOP, nonreducing disc displacement, and TMJ pain, except that contracture does not usually hurt unless the muscle is stretched beyond the point of resistance.[61]

Hypertrophy

Most commonly, it is a painless condition associated with enlargement in the masticatory muscle possibly related to overuse, familial, genetic, or chronic bracing of muscles.[61]

MASTICATORY MUSCLE PAIN ATTRIBUTED TO SYSTEMIC/CENTRAL PAIN DISORDERS
Fibromyalgia

The diffuse chronic widespread pain, hyperalgesia, and allodynia in FM have been previously hypothesized to be due to central mechanisms. However, recently it is hypothesized that the condition may be a spectrum secondary to multiple potential mechanisms with varying degrees of peripheral and central components across the spectrum of presentations. The mechanisms may include biological amplification of sensory pain inputs, affective components of pain processing, alterations in neurotransmitters and their receptors, enhanced connections with the insula in the resting state, reduced connectivity among antinociceptive areas, augmented pain processing, altered immunologic, inflammatory mechanisms, and defective pain modulation in descending inhibitory systems.[71] Patients with TMD may share many features with FM. Both are characterized by musculoskeletal pain. Although FM diagnosis generally requires more locations than just the jaw, the American College of Rheumatology Preliminary Diagnostic Criteria for FM allows for as few as 3 locations (the right jaw, left jaw, and neck, for example), so long as other symptoms are more severe or abundant. Those other symptoms include fatigue, waking unrefreshed, muscle weakness, depression, nervousness, and so forth; such symptoms are nonspecific and may occur in patients with TMD. Patients with TMD also may have pains elsewhere in the body, further increasing the chance of confusing TMD for FM or vice versa. The use of a validated FM diagnostic is the most certain way to achieve an accurate diagnosis.[72]

HEADACHES

Headache has been reported in many TMDs cases, but the relationship between these 2 conditions is still controversial.[3] A study in the US population reported that 61.3% of patients with orofacial pain reported headaches with migraine (with or without aura) specifically affecting 38% of this population,[73] and specifically 72.7% of patients with TMD reported headaches.[74] A 5-year prospective study reported that in patients with migraine and tension-type headaches (TTHs), prevalence and frequency of headaches were strong indicators for the development of TMD. Multiple mechanisms including genetics, trigeminocervical sensitization, and biopsychosocial and environmental factors have been hypothesized to play a role.[29]

Tension-Type Headache

TTH is a primary headache characterized by bilateral mild or moderate pressing or tightening pain, which is not worsened by routine physical activity. Because TTH often overlaps with the temporalis region, feels as a physical pressure, lacks nausea and vomiting, and often lacks photophobia and phonophobia,[6] it at times is confused with temporalis MOP. Differentiation is made by the fact that temporalis MOP is aggravated by palpation and jaw function.[3,62]

Migraine Headache

Migraine headache is a primary headache characterized by moderate-to-severe unilateral pulsating pain aggravated by routine physical activity, as well as nausea, vomiting, photophobia, and/or phonophobia.[75] Because migraine headaches may overlap with the temporalis region and are worsened with physical activity, migraine patients are more likely to have TMD, and TMD and migraine headaches can trigger or aggravate each other,[76,77] migraines are sometimes confused with temporalis MOP.

However, the associated signs of nausea, vomiting, photophobia, and phonophobia, as well as the response to migraine-specific medications, help the clinician recognize migraine headaches. The absence of pain with jaw function and palpation of the temporalis also suggest migraine headaches over temporalis MOP.

CORONOID HYPERPLASIA

An abnormal enlargement of the coronoid process should be considered as a TMD condition that lies in the subcategory of associated structures.[61]

PERSISTENT IDIOPATHIC FACIAL PAIN

Persistent idiopathic facial pain is characterized by poorly localized dull, aching, or nagging pain that does not follow the distribution of a peripheral nerve. The pain can feel deep and can be aggravated by stress. When the location overlaps masticatory muscles and/or the TMJ, this fairly nonspecific pain condition can seem to be a TMD. The main points of differentiation are the aggravation of TMD by palpation and/or jaw function.[62]

CLINICAL IMPLICATIONS

Although the complexity of the etiopathogenic domains may seem overwhelming, there are significant clinical implications in terms of diagnosis and management. First and foremost, the incorporation of validated questionnaires, screening tools, or checklists assessing risk factors may help in the identification of the patient population at risk for developing these conditions and enable the clustering of patients. Risk factors are a significant contributor to the development of TMDs. Identification and addressing these risk factors may result in a substantial reduction in the incident, and recurrent TMDs curtailing and addressing the deleterious oral parafunctional risk factors and enhancing positive modifying factors are crucial to success; this may also be an effective way to prevent the development of incident TMD and reduce dependence on health care resources. In addition to promoting features for peripheral management; emphasis may also be placed on improving general health outcomes and addressing health and pain comorbidities. Traditionally home care instructions have included local measures to provide pain relief. Emphasis on general health care measures may help in addressing additional comorbidities and COPCs, thus improving general health. The distinction between acute, chronic, single versus recurrent, persistent pain and regional/localized versus widespread TMD and the etiopathological mechanism is critical to developing a management or treatment strategies. Identification of distinct pathophysiological pathways, biopsychosocial risk factors, and pain profiling in patients may help in developing clusters of individual patients, predict prognosis, and use precision medicine to enhance success rates of management. Current research suggests that simple therapy may suffice in patients without significant psychological symptoms, whereas multimodal, interdisciplinary management may be required for complex patients with major psychological risk factors. Identifying the complexity may form a platform for the clinician to initiate discussion and patient education for interdisciplinary management. Hence, it is also important to follow the progression of individual parameters across various time points in an individual to assess the development of systemic confounders affecting treatment prognosis and management. Finally, the identification of pathophysiological mechanisms may enable targeted pharmacologic interventions. For instance, if peripheral factors predominate, topical and pharmacologic medications targeting peripheral sensitization mediators may be more effective, whereas in chronic conditions centrally acting medications may be required.

CLINICS CARE POINTS

- The understanding of peripherally and centrally mediated pain can better help manage patients. Referred pain from non-odontogenic regions can reflect as odontogenic pain.

DISCLOSURE

The authors have nothing to disclose.

REFERENCES

1. Slade GD, Ohrbach R, Greenspan JD, et al. Painful temporomandibular disorder: decade of discovery from OPERA studies. J Dent Res 2016;95(10):1084–92.
2. Slade GD, Bair E, Greenspan JD, et al. Signs and symptoms of first-onset TMD and sociodemographic predictors of its development: the OPPERA prospective cohort study. J Pain 2013;14(12 Suppl):T20–32 e1-3.
3. Schiffman E, Ohrbach R, Trueloveet E, et al. Diagnostic Criteria for Temporomandibular Disorders (DC/TMD) for Clinical and Research Applications: recommendations of the International RDC/TMD Consortium Network* and Orofacial Pain Special Interest Groupdagger. J Oral Facial Pain Headache 2014;28(1):6–27.
4. Rongo R, Ekberg E, Nilsson I, et al. Diagnostic criteria for temporomandibular disorders (DC/TMD) for children and adolescents: An international Delphi study-Part 1-Development of Axis I. J Oral Rehabil 2021;48(7):836–45.
5. Slade GD, Fillingim R, Sanders A, et al. Summary of findings from the OPPERA prospective cohort study of incidence of first-onset temporomandibular disorder: implications and future directions. J Pain 2013;14(12 Suppl):T116–24.
6. Manfredini D, Lombardo L, Siciliani G. Temporomandibular disorders and dental occlusion. A systematic review of association studies: end of an era? J Oral Rehabil 2017;44(11):908–23.
7. Gesch D, Bernhardt O, Kirbschus A. Association of malocclusion and functional occlusion with temporomandibular disorders (TMD) in adults: a systematic review of population-based studies. Quintessence Int 2004;35(3):211–21.
8. Kalladka M, Young A, Thomas D, et al. The relation of temporomandibular disorders and dental occlusion: a narrative review. Quintessence Int 2022;53(5):450–9.
9. Bair E, Ohrbach R, Fillingim R, et al. Multivariable modeling of phenotypic risk factors for first-onset TMD: the OPPERA prospective cohort study. J Pain 2013;14(12 Suppl):T102–15.
10. Moin Anwer HM, Albagieh H, Kalladka M, et al. The role of the dentist in the diagnosis and management of pediatric obstructive sleep apnea. Saudi Dent J 2021;33(7):424–33.
11. Ozasa K, Nishihara C, Watanabe K, et al. Somatosensory profile of a patient with mixed connective tissue disease and Sjogren syndrome. J Am Dent Assoc 2020;151(2):145–51.
12. Sanders AE, Slade G, Bair E, et al. General health status and incidence of first-onset temporomandibular disorder: the OPPERA prospective cohort study. J Pain 2013;14(12 Suppl):T51–62.

13. Gaynor SM, Fillingim R, Zolnounet D, et al. Association of Hormonal Contraceptive Use with Headache and Temporomandibular Pain: The OPPERA Study. J Oral Facial Pain Headache 2021;35(2):105–12.
14. Markiewicz MR, Ohrbach R, McCall WD Jr. Oral behaviors checklist: reliability of performance in targeted waking-state behaviors. J Orofac Pain 2006;20(4): 306–16.
15. Ohrbach R, Bair E, Fillingim R, Gonzalez Y, et al. Clinical orofacial characteristics associated with risk of first-onset TMD: the OPPERA prospective cohort study. J Pain 2013;14(12 Suppl):T33–50.
16. Sharma S, Wactawski-Wende J, LaMonte M, et al. Incident injury is strongly associated with subsequent incident temporomandibular disorder: results from the OPPERA study. Pain 2019;160(7):1551–61.
17. Slade GD, Sanders A, Ohrbach R, et al. Pressure pain thresholds fluctuate with, but do not usefully predict, the clinical course of painful temporomandibular disorder. Pain 2014;155(10):2134–43.
18. Sanders AE, Essick G, Fillingim R, et al. Sleep apnea symptoms and risk of temporomandibular disorder: OPPERA cohort. J Dent Res 2013;92(7 Suppl):70S.
19. Sanders AE, Akinkugbe A, Fillingimet R, et al. Causal mediation in the development of painful temporomandibular disorder. J Pain 2017;18(4):428–36.
20. Fillingim RB, Ohrbach R, Greenspan J, et al. Psychological factors associated with development of TMD: the OPPERA prospective cohort study. J Pain 2013; 14(12 Suppl):T75–90.
21. Aggarwal VR, Macfarlane G, Farragher T, et al. Risk factors for onset of chronic oro-facial pain–results of the North Cheshire oro-facial pain prospective population study. Pain 2010;149(2):354–9.
22. Dunn KM, Jordan K, Mancl L, et al. Trajectories of pain in adolescents: a prospective cohort study. Pain 2011;152(1):66–73.
23. LeResche L, Mancl L, Drangsholt M, et al. Predictors of onset of facial pain and temporomandibular disorders in early adolescence. Pain 2007;129(3):269–78.
24. Fillingim RB, Ohrbach R, Greenspan J, et al. Associations of psychologic factors with multiple chronic overlapping pain conditions. J Oral Facial Pain Headache 2020;34:s85–100.
25. Euteneuer F, Schwarz M, Hennings A, et al. Psychobiological aspects of somatization syndromes: contributions of inflammatory cytokines and neopterin. Psychiatry Res 2012;195(1–2):60–5.
26. Maes M. Inflammatory and oxidative and nitrosative stress pathways underpinning chronic fatigue, somatization and psychosomatic symptoms. Curr Opin Psychiatry 2009;22(1):75–83.
27. Fillingim RB, Slade G, Greenspan J, et al. Long-term changes in biopsychosocial characteristics related to temporomandibular disorder: findings from the OPPERA study. Pain 2018;159(11):2403–13.
28. Smith SB, Mir E, Blair E, et al. Genetic variants associated with development of TMD and its intermediate phenotypes: the genetic architecture of TMD in the OPPERA prospective cohort study. J Pain 2013;14(12 Suppl):T91–101 e1-3.
29. Tchivileva IE, Ohrbach R, Fillingim R, et al. Temporal change in headache and its contribution to the risk of developing firstonset temporomandibular disorder in the Orofacial Pain: Prospective Evaluation and Risk Assessment (OPPERA) study. Pain 2017;158(1):120–9.
30. Slade GD, Rosen J, Ohrbach R, et al. Anatomical selectivity in overlap of chronic facial and bodily pain. Pain Rep 2019;4(3):e729.

31. Jensen R. Mechanisms of spontaneous tension-type headaches: an analysis of tenderness, pain thresholds and EMG. Pain 1996;64(2):251–6.

32. Morch CD, Hu J, Arendt-Nielsen L, et al. Convergence of cutaneous, musculoskeletal, dural and visceral afferents onto nociceptive neurons in the first cervical dorsal horn. Eur J Neurosci 2007;26(1):142–54.

33. Rodriguez E, Sakurai K, Xu J, et al. A craniofacial-specific monosynaptic circuit enables heightened affective pain. Nat Neurosci 2017;20(12):1734–43.

34. Scholz J, Woolf CJ. The neuropathic pain triad: neurons, immune cells and glia. Nat Neurosci 2007;10(11):1361–8.

35. Kaneyama K, Segami N, Sun W, et al. Analysis of tumor necrosis factor-alpha, interleukin-6, interleukin-1beta, soluble tumor necrosis factor receptors I and II, interleukin-6 soluble receptor, interleukin-1 soluble receptor type II, interleukin-1 receptor antagonist, and protein in the synovial fluid of patients with temporomandibular joint disorders. Oral Surg Oral Med Oral Pathol Oral Radiol Endod 2005; 99(3):276–84.

36. Lee JK, Cho YS, Song SI. Relationship of synovial tumor necrosis factor alpha and interleukin 6 to temporomandibular disorder. J Oral Maxillofac Surg 2010; 68(5):1064–8.

37. Harmon JB, Sanders A, Wilder R, et al. Circulating omentin-1 and chronic painful temporomandibular disorders. J Oral Facial Pain Headache 2016;30(3):203–9.

38. Slade GD, Conrad M, Diatchenko L, et al. Cytokine biomarkers and chronic pain: association of genes, transcription, and circulating proteins with temporomandibular disorders and widespread palpation tenderness. Pain 2011;152(12): 2802–12.

39. Cheng JK, Ji RR. Intracellular signaling in primary sensory neurons and persistent pain. Neurochem Res 2008;33(10):1970–8.

40. Zhang JM, An J. , Cytokines, inflammation, and pain. Int Anesthesiol Clin 2007; 45(2):27–37.

41. Kaneyama K, Segami N, Nishimura M, et al. Importance of proinflammatory cytokines in synovial fluid from 121 joints with temporomandibular disorders. Br J Oral Maxillofac Surg 2002;40(5):418–23.

42. Takahashi T, Kondoh T, Fukuda M, et al. Proinflammatory cytokines detectable in synovial fluids from patients with temporomandibular disorders. Oral Surg Oral Med Oral Pathol Oral Radiol Endod 1998;85(2):135–41.

43. Eliav E, Benoliel R, Herzberg H, et al. The role of IL-6 and IL-1beta in painful perineural inflammatory neuritis. Brain Behav Immun 2009;23(4):474–84.

44. Kopp S. Neuroendocrine, immune, and local responses related to temporomandibular disorders. J Orofac Pain 2001;15(1):9–28.

45. Maixner W, Diatchenko L, Dubner R, et al. Orofacial pain prospective evaluation and risk assessment study–the OPPERA study. J Pain 2011;12(11 Suppl): T4–11 e1-2.

46. Khan J, Wang Q, Ren Y, et al. Exercise induced hypoalgesia profile in rats is associated with IL-10 and IL-1 beta levels and pain severity following nerve injury. Cytokine 2021;143:155540.

47. Korczeniewska OA, Kuo F, Huang C, et al. Genetic variation in catechol-O-methyltransferase is associated with individual differences in conditioned pain modulation in healthy subjects. J Gene Med 2021;23(11):e3374.

48. Bair E, Gaynor S, Slade G, et al. Identification of clusters of individuals relevant to temporomandibular disorders and other chronic pain conditions: the OPPERA study. Pain 2016;157(6):1266–78.

49. Young A, Gallia S, Ryan J, et al. Diagnostic tool using the diagnostic criteria for temporomandibular disorders: a randomized crossover-controlled, double-blinded, two-center study. J Oral Facial Pain Headache 2021;35(3):241–52.

50. Ahmad M, Schiffman EL. Temporomandibular joint disorders and orofacial pain. Dent Clin North Am 2016;60(1):105–24.

51. Manfredini D. Etiopathogenesis of disk displacement of the temporomandibular joint: a review of the mechanisms. Indian J Dent Res 2009;20(2):212–21.

52. Wang ZH, Zhao YP, Ma XC. Ankylosis of temporomandibular joint caused by psoriatic arthritis: a report of four cases with literature review. Chin J Dent Res 2014; 17(1):49–55.

53. Kobayashi R, Utsunomiya T, Yamamoto H, et al. Ankylosis of the temporomandibular joint caused by rheumatoid arthritis: a pathological study and review. J Oral Sci 2001;43(2):97–101.

54. Herford AS, Boyne PJ. Ankylosis of the jaw in a patient with fibrodysplasia ossificans progressiva. Oral Surg Oral Med Oral Pathol Oral Radiol Endod 2003; 96(6):680–4.

55. Rongo R, Alstergren P, Ammendola L, et al. Temporomandibular joint damage in juvenile idiopathic arthritis: diagnostic validity of diagnostic criteria for temporomandibular disorders. J Oral Rehabil 2019;46(5):450–9.

56. Long X. The relationship between temporomandibular joint ankylosis and condylar fractures. Chin J Dent Res 2012;15(1):17–20.

57. Abrahamsson H, Eriksson L, Abrahamsson P, et al. Treatment of temporomandibular joint luxation: a systematic literature review. Clin Oral Investig 2020;24(1): 61–70.

58. Muto T, Kawakami J, Kanazawa M, et al. Development and histologic characteristics of synovitis induced by trauma in the rat temporomandibular joint. Int J Oral Maxillofac Surg 1998;27(6):470–5.

59. Dijkstra PU, Kropmans TJ, Stegenga B. The association between generalized joint hypermobility and temporomandibular joint disorders: a systematic review. J Dent Res 2002;81(3):158–63.

60. Kalladka M, Quek S, Heir G, et al. Temporomandibular joint osteoarthritis: diagnosis and long-term conservative management: a topic review. J Indian Prosthodont Soc 2014;14(1):6–15.

61. Peck CC, Goulet J-P, Lobbezoo F, et al. Expanding the taxonomy of the diagnostic criteria for temporomandibular disorders. J Oral Rehabil 2014;41(1):2–23.

62. International Classification of Orofacial Pain, 1st edition (ICOP). Cephalalgia Int J Headache 2020;40(2):129–221.

63. Nicolielo LFP, Jacobs R, Albdour E, et al. Is oestrogen associated with mandibular condylar resorption? A systematic review. Int J Oral Maxillofac Surg 2017; 46(11):1394–402.

64. Ivask O, Leibur E, Voog-Oras U. Synovial chondromatosis in the temporomandibular joint: case report with review of the literature. Stomatologija 2015;17(3): 97–101.

65. Robinson D, Hasharoni A, Cohen N, et al. Fibroblast growth factor receptor-3 as a marker for precartilaginous stem cells. Clin Orthop Relat Res 1999;367(Suppl): S163–75.

66. Fujita S, Iizuka T, Yoshida H, et al. Transforming growth factor and tenascin in synovial chondromatosis of the temporomandibular joint. Report of a case. Int J Oral Maxillofac Surg 1997;26(4):258–9.

67. Li Y, Zhou Y, Wang Y, et al. Synovial macrophages in cartilage destruction and regeneration-lessons learnt from osteoarthritis and synovial chondromatosis. Biomed Mater 2021;17(1).
68. Ferguson M. Rhinosinusitis in oral medicine and dentistry. Aust Dent J 2014; 59(3):289–95.
69. Williams JW, Simel DL. Does this patient have sinusitis? Diagnosing acute sinusitis by history and physical examination. JAMA 1993;270(10):1242–6.
70. Shivhare P, Shankarnarayan L, Usha, et al. Condylar aplasia and hypoplasia: a rare case. Case Rep Dent 2013;2013:745602.
71. Kalladka M, Young A, Khan J. Myofascial pain in temporomandibular disorders: Updates on etiopathogenesis and management. J Bodyw Mov Ther 2021;28: 104–13.
72. Wolfe F, Clauw DJ, Fitzcharles MA, et al. The American College of Rheumatology preliminary diagnostic criteria for fibromyalgia and measurement of symptom severity. Arthritis Care Res 2010;62(5):600–10.
73. Sluka KA, Clauw DJ. Neurobiology of fibromyalgia and chronic widespread pain. Neuroscience 2016;338:114–29.
74. Dando WE, Branch MA, Maye JP. Headache disability in orofacial pain patients. Headache 2006;46(2):322–6.
75. Olesen J. International classification of headache disorders. Lancet Neurol 2018; 17(5):396–7.
76. Teruel A, Romero-Reyes M. Interplay of oral, mandibular, and facial disorders and migraine. Curr Pain Headache Rep 2022;26(7):517–23.
77. Covert L, Mater HV, Hechler BL. Comprehensive management of rheumatic diseases affecting the temporomandibular joint. Diagnostics (Basel) 2021;11(3).

Systemic Factors in Temporomandibular Disorder Pain

Davis C. Thomas, BDS, DDS, MSD, MSc Med, MSc[a,b,*],
Eli Eliav, DMD, MSc, PhD[c], Antonio Romero Garcia, DDS, PhD, MSc[d],
Mahnaz Fatahzadeh, DMD, MSD[e]

KEYWORDS

- Temporomandibular joint disorder • TMJ • TMD • Systemic factors • Fibromyalgia
- Arthritis • Autoimmune • Musculoskeletal pain

KEY POINTS

- The effect of systemic factors affecting temporomandibular disorder (TMD) pain is a crucial concept for the treating physician to understand for the effective management of TMD pain.
- In the absence of delineation of the systemic factors that may condition the patient's experience of TMD pain, the clinician–patient team may most likely encounter the problem of suboptimal management of pain.
- A complete discussion of the numerous systemic factors that affect TMD pain experience is well beyond the scope of any single article. It is up to pain education programs, and individual clinicians, to educate the medical community regarding the significance of managing TMD pain, through effective management of the systemic condition.
- The dental clinician and orofacial pain specialist must be aware of basic and more advanced appropriate laboratory tests to be ordered when conditioning systemic factors affecting TMD pain are suspected. This will help facilitate prompt appropriate referral to succinct involved specialties.
- Any clinician attempting to manage TMD pain must be familiar with the possible interplay between multiple systemic factors and possible medications, as it affects the patient's experience of pain.

[a] Department of Diagnostic Sciences, Rutgers School of Dental Medicine, 110 Bergen Street, Newark, NJ 07103, USA; [b] Eastman Institute of Oral Health, Rochester, NY, USA; [c] Eastman Institute for Oral Health, University of Rochester Medical Center, 625 Elmwood Avenue, Rochester, NY 14620, USA; [d] CranioClinic, Valencia and Dental Sleep Solutions, Plaza San Agustin, Portal C, Piso 2, Puerta 2, Valencia 46002, Spain; [e] Division of Oral Medicine, Department of Oral Medicine, Rutgers School of Dental Medicine, 110 Bergen Street, Newark, NJ 07103, USA
* Corresponding author.
E-mail address: davisct1@gmail.com

Dent Clin N Am 67 (2023) 281–298
https://doi.org/10.1016/j.cden.2022.10.002
0011-8532/23/© 2022 Elsevier Inc. All rights reserved.

dental.theclinics.com

INTRODUCTION

Temporomandibular disorders (TMD) are considered the second most prevalent painful musculoskeletal condition (second to chronic low back pain), and affects between 6% and 12% of the general population.[1] It is also proposed that approximately 15% of this population develop chronic TMD.[1] TMD pain is considered the most common cause of nondental orofacial pain.[2,3] Pain is a very subjective phenomenon. A higher prevalence of chronic pain and high-impact chronic pain exists among US women.[4] The experience of pain anywhere in the body is conceivably influenced significantly by systemic factors, including, but not limited to, genetics, gender, nutritional status, metabolic disorders, psychological factors, immunologic conditions, endocrine disorders, sleep disorders, and more recently, COVID-19 infection. It follows that, the same would be true of TMD and TMD pain as well. Systemic factors have a profound influence on pain threshold, pain sensitivity and the overall experience of pain. A single systemic factor such as anemia[5–7] or vitamin D deficiency[8,9] can by itself condition the patient's experience of pain significantly, directly or indirectly, or both. When multiple systemic factors are figured in, this scenario becomes much more complex, both for the patient with TMD and the clinician.

A comprehensive discussion of all the systemic factors that affect TMD and TMD pain is well beyond the purview of a single article such as this one. This manuscript discusses the most cardinal factors that may affect the experience of pain in a patient with TMD, within the limitations of a single article. Conceivably, the management of the systemic factor/s that condition the patient's pain experience is crucial to achieving optimal pain control in TMD. The thought process that went into the creation of such an article stemmed from several interesting scientific queries and observations. Being that the most prevalent orofacial pain is TMD pain,[1] and the most prevalent of the TMD pain is myalgia and myofascial pain,[10,11] the questions are "what is the most common cause of muscle pain?"; "what are the common diagnoses that are associated with myalgia?"; "what are the common diseases with arthralgia?"; and "What converts a chronic bruxer 'grinding' painlessly for several years to now complaining of pain in the masticatory musculature?". When a patient presents to a dentist including an orofacial pain specialist with a complaint of "I grind my teeth and I have pain"—how many clinicians routinely look for other sites of pain, global pain, or systemic conditions that may have predisposed the patient to pain?". Based on available literature, we discuss the most important systemic factors that may affect the pain experience of a patient with TMD.

Arthritis

It is well known that the types of arthritis that affects temporomandibular joint (TMJ) and associated structures are rheumatoid arthritis (RA), osteoarthritis (OA), and psoriatic arthritis (PsA), among others. RA affects approximately 1.5% of the general population.[12] Considering this prevalence in the general population, and the fact that most of the patients presenting to an orofacial pain clinician likely are a different pool of patients already in pain, it follows that the prevalence/incidence of RA in patients with TMD pain may actually be much higher. The differentiation between the 3 major types of systemic arthritis, namely RA, OA, and PsA can be clinically difficult. Pain may be the common factor for all the 3 types of arthritis. It must be noted that contrary to the popular thought that RA afflicts the mineralized structures of the joints, the entity robustly affects both the mineralized and the nonmineralized tissues of the body in general, and the joints in particular. RA affects soft tissues such as muscles, ligaments and tendons associated with the TMJ.[12] OA affects primarily the larger and load-bearing joints. It must be noted that there are systemic symptoms associated with OA as well.[13,14]

For the purpose of this review, we have taken PsA as the prototype to discuss the features of the entity. More than 50% of patients with RA show signs and symptoms of TMJ involvement.[15] By and large, the basis of joint pain in RA is the resultant ligamental laxity, tendinal and ligamental disintegration, and subsequent joint destruction.[12] These also form the foundation for bony erosions, bone and joint deformities, impaired muscle and joint function, and much reduced quality of life (QoL) in these patients. A comparison of these 3 entities is presented in **Table 1**.

Psoriatic Arthritis: a Prototype for Temporomandibular Joint Arthritides

The authors chose PsA as a prototype for arthritides affecting the TMJ, due to the robust features it has, as a systemic chronic inflammatory rheumatologic condition, in patients with psoriasis.[16–18] We took a novel approach and selected PsA due to the unique combination it presents of systemic and local effects on the patient, and have attempted to compare and contrast with the other arthritic entities wherever possible. The readers must be aware that PsA is not the most prevalent arthritic affliction of the TMJ. In most of those with PsA (60%–80%), skin symptoms precede the onset of arthralgia[16,19,20] but 15% to 20% of individuals experience rheumatological symptomatology prior to[16,20], or simultaneous with the skin manifestations.[16,19,20] There are several arthritic entities including RA, OA, gouty arthritis, and other autoimmune conditions that can have similar clinical features. The readers are recommended to refer to the articles referenced in this manuscript for a detailed description of other types of arthritides that affect the TMJ.

The worldwide prevalence of PsA varies depending on the population studied; however, a recent systematic review estimates this condition affects 1 in 4 individuals with psoriasis.[21] According to the National Psoriasis Foundation, 30% of Americans with psoriasis could have PsA.[22] The condition more often affects whites and adults 30 to 55 years of age with no gender predilection.[17] PsA typically has an insidious onset and a progressive course with periodic flares and remissions in symptoms.[17] This is much similar to the presentation of RA and OA.[12] Patients may experience constitutional symptoms such as fever, fatigue, malaise, and myalgia. This necessitates to differentiate from other rheumatologic disorders, such as RA and gout, with similar features. In most patients (95%), PsA could affect peripheral joints of hands, elbows, shoulders, knees, ankles, and toes.[23] A multifactorial cause contributes to the autoimmune inflammatory nature of tissue damage seen in both psoriasis and PsA.[20,23] There may be a familial/genetic predisposition, similar to RA, OA, and gouty arthritis.[24,25]

The TMJ could be affected in PsA,[16,19] and there have been reports of TMJ arthropathy as the first sign of PsA.[19] Nevertheless, the prevalence of TMJ disease as a manifestation of PsA has not been systematically studied, and the general consensus is that PsA rarely affects TMJ.[16–18,22] However, when present, the TMD symptoms including pain are very much similar to those of other afflictions of the TMJ such as RA and painful OA. Depending on the severity, signs and symptoms of psoriatic TMJ involvement could include jaw stiffness, pain during function, preauricular swelling, TMJ crepitation, earache, tenderness of joint and masticatory muscles upon palpation, occlusal derangement as well as reduced range of motion, and interincisal opening.[17] Both TMJ symptomatology and potential disability could adversely affect the QoL and psychological well-being in those affected.[18,23] Radiographic evidence of TMJ damage in PsA include erosion of cortical outline, flattening of condylar head, narrowing of joint space, articular effusion, and formation of calcified spicules and osteophytes.[16,23,26,27] Once again, these are very similar to the clinical and

Table 1
Comparison of salient features of psoriatic, rheumatoid, and osteoarthritis

	Psoriatic Arthritis	Rheumatoid Arthritis	Osteoarthritis
Diagnostic criteria	2006 CASPAR criteria • Evidence of psoriasis (current/former/family history) • Dactylitis • Juxta-articular new-bone formation • RF negativity • Nail dystrophy	2010 ACR/EULAR criteria • Synovitis in > 1 joint • No alternative diagnosis • Number of involved joints • RF ± anti-CCP +/− • Elevated ESR or CRP • Symptoms for >6 wk	ACR criteria (separate for hip/knee/hand) (modified from ACR 2010) Using history, physical examination, laboratory findings • Local pain • ESR less than ACR specified value • Limitation of function • RF less than the varied ACR-determined values • Radiographic findings
Patterns of arthropathy	• Asymmetric oligoarticular arthritis • Symmetric polyarthritis • Possible distal interphalangeal arthropathy • Arthritis mutilans • Spondylitis ± sacroiliitis	• Symmetric polyarthritis (fingers, wrists) • Metacarpophalangeal (MCP) and proximal interphalangeal (PIP) arthropathy • Spondylitis limited to cervical spine • No sacroiliitis	• Abnormal remodeling of subchondral bone • Chondrocyte apoptosis • Upregulated catabolic enzymes
Extra-articular findings	• Current or prior cutaneous lesions of psoriasis or family history of psoriasis • Nail dystrophy (onycholysis, pitting, hyperkeratosis, splinter hemorrhage) • Uveitis, conjunctivitis, iritis • Rare subcutaneous nodules • Synovitis limited to flexor tendon sheaths	• No cutaneous lesions • Common subcutaneous nodules • No nail involvement • Vasculitis • Scleritis, episcleritis (not uveitis) • Synovitis involving both flexor and extensor tendon sheaths	• None • Other visceral organs are not affected

	Column 1	Column 2	Column 3
Serologic findings	• RF negative • Anti-CCP negative • HLA-B27 negative (except for axial PsA)	• RF positive (in most patients) • Anti-CCP positive • HLA-B27 negative • Elevated ESR (<100) • Elevated C-reactive protein (CRP) • Positive ANA (30%)	• RF: Negative • ESR: Normal • CRP: Normal • SERUM ANA, CRP, ESR increases with age
Clinical findings in TMJ arthropathy	• Periauricular pain and swelling • Jaw deviation on opening and closure • Occlusal derangement • Reduced range of motion • Joint crepitus	• Reduced range of motion • Joint crepitus	• Deterioration of cartilage • Abnormal remodeling of the joint • Pain • Joint stiffness • Limited mouth opening • Hypersensitivity to cold • Crepitus • Absence of joint warmth • Occlusal changes
Radiographic findings	• Erosion of condylar cortical margins (deplaned condylar head) • Minimal juxta-articular osteopenia • Subchondral osteolysis • Decreased joint space • Articular effusion • Osteophytic spurs • Fibrosis in advanced disease • Ankylosis is uncommon	• Erosion of condylar cortical margins (deplaned condylar head) • Juxta-articular osteopenia • Subchondral osteolysis • Decreased joint space • Articular effusion • Uncommon osteophytic spurs • Ankylosis is rare	• Erosion • Flattening • Sclerosis • Subcortical cysts • Osteophytes • Deformity

Abbreviations: ACR, American College of Rheumatology; ANA, antinuclear antibodies; Anti-CCP, Anti-cyclic citrullinated peptide; CRP, C-reactive protein; ESR, erythrocyte sedimentation rate; RF, rheumatoid factor.
Table content based on references.[16,17,23,24,26,28,30]

radiographic features of the other arthritides mentioned previously.[12] Much similar to the other arthritides, management of arthropathy including TMJ in PsA is not curative, but lifelong, and aimed at controlling symptoms, improving function and preventing further joint damage.[12,17,18,23,28]

Management of any arthritidic entities of the TMJ is tailored to the patient's age, severity of symptoms and overall health, particularly in the presence of extra-articular manifestations. A holistic approach includes health education (reassurance, joint rest, soft diet, minimal mouth opening, warm compresses for spastic muscles, stress-reduction), physical therapy,[17,18,23,29] occlusal splints (to reduce joint pain and swelling, management of nocturnal parafunction)[17,18,23] intra-articular glucocorticoid injections to relieve synovitis,[17,18,28] analgesics such as non-steroidal anti-inflammatory drugs (NSAIDs),[17,23,28] and conventional disease-modifying antirheumatic drugs (DMARDs) including biologic agents.[17,28,30] When indicated, early pharmacologic intervention is warranted to prevent further joint damage.[28]

Patients with refractory disease may be considered for interventions such as arthroscopy, arthrocentesis, surgery, or joint replacement.[17,18,23,30] Although studies indicate higher frequency and severity of TMD signs and symptoms in patients with PsA compared with healthy individuals,[18,31,32] the reported cases of TMJ arthropathy remains low.[33] One explanation is that TMJ is often overlooked in the overall assessment of patients by rheumatologists,[16,34] and this omission could lead to underrecognition of TMJ involvement.[17] Patients with PsA could also have late onset of symptoms or remain symptom-free despite significant joint destruction.[28] Therefore, in the absence of imaging, TMJ arthropathy could be missed. In contrast, RA and OA have marked changes in the joint especially when chronic.[12] Evaluation of patients with new onset of TMJ signs and symptoms by dental providers should include a thorough medical history and review of systems for constitutional symptoms, ophthalmologic problems and lesions of integumentary system (skin and nails) as well as muscular weakness, backache, arthralgia and joint dysfunction elsewhere in the body.[18,28] Discovery of TMJ involvement in rheumatologic patients should be communicated to the patient's physician to allow necessary modifications to pharmacologic management.[18]

Autoimmune Rheumatological Diseases

Many rheumatological diseases have an autoimmune etiopathology and have been shown to be the cause of global pain, central sensitization states, and chronic pain.[35,36] Conceivably, these entities can have profound effects on the head and neck, and TMD pain as well. It must be noted that there may be considerable overlap between autoimmune/rheumatological diseases and other systemic conditions. Therefore, a crystal-clear delineation between various entities may not be practical. Systemic lupus erythematosus (SLE) is seen as the poster child for affliction of the systems in the rheumatology literature.[12] With a much higher prevalence of RA in the general population, the American College of Rheumatology's guidelines dictate that RA should be considered as a rule out when a single joint swelling and pain is manifested in a patient.[37] Widespread pain is reported approximately by 40% of SLE patients and musculoskeletal involvement is responsible for significant reduction in QoL in these patients.[38] TMJ involvement in SLE has been reported with a prevalence of 0.25% and in RA with a prevalence of 0.5% to 1%.[12]

The other entities that may need to be ruled out if TMD presents with global pain and other systemic symptoms are scleroderma, Sjogren's, Raynaud's, gout, reactive arthritis, and polymyalgia rheumatica (PMR).[39,40] The most common complaints occurring with approximately 90% of SLE patients are those related to inflammatory arthralgia and nonerosive nondeforming arthritis.[38] Lupus headache is reported in approximate average of 50% of SLE patients, with fibromyalgia coexisting in 30% of these patients.[41] Myalgia of muscles of mastication, the neck and the shoulder and a feeling of "stuck jaw" and tinnitus are the most common TMD symptoms in SLE patients.[42]

Diet and Nutrition

Many nutritional and dietary factors have been proposed to be associated with pain in general, and TMD pain in particular. These include vitamins, micronutrients and macronutrients, and electrolytes.[7,43] On the contrary, there have been publications quoting studies that apparently showed that many nutritional factors do not have a role in TMD pain.[44] Vitamin D has been shown in studies to reduce pain scores.[45,46] It must be noted that several mechanisms have been proposed for the role of Vitamin D in sleep and in pain.[47] Vitamin D deficiency and low consumption of calcium were found to be associated with sleep-related bruxism (SRB), anxiety, and depression, entities that are known to be associated with TMD and TMD pain.[48] There is some evidence in the current literature that the nature of the diet and lack of dietary quality can affect chronic musculoskeletal pain.[49] The role of diet and nutrition is discussed elsewhere in a separate chapter titled "Diet and Nutritional factors in TMD?" in this special edition.

Infections

In this world of constantly changing newer infections, a few of them merit mention when considering their possible relationship with chronic pain such as that associated with TMD. The COVID-19 pandemic/affliction has currently jumped to the top of this list. The other worth-mentioning infections include, but not limited to, Epstein Barr virus (EBV), Cytomegalovirus (CMV), and Lyme disease (LD).

LD is considered a vector-borne disease, the causative organism being the bacterium *Borrelia burgdorferi*. The disease is transmitted by ticks.[50,51] Lyme patients have reported neck and back pain.[52] Lyme patients have a very high incidence of myofascial pain.[53] It has been proposed that TMD pain is more in bruxers with LD.[54] In addition, complaints of headache, disturbed sleep, global myalgia, impaired cognitive function, fatigue, paresthesias, and weakness have been reported in chronic Lyme.[55,56] According to the current Centers for Disease Control (CDC) website, as of 2019, the prevalence and incidence of Lyme is the highest in the northeast of the United States.

CMV and EBV are both associated with infectious mononucleosis, and highly prevalent in the general population.[57,58] Primary CMV infection has been shown to be associated with generalized malaise and myalgia in approximately 60% to 70% of immunocompetent patients.[59] New daily persistent headache was shown in approximately 10% of CMV-positive patients.[60,61] EBV has been associated with autoimmune diseases such as multiple sclerosis.[62–64] EBV infection has also shown to be associated with polyarthralgia, many a times mimicking the joint pain of RA.[65] The clinician attempting to manage TMD pain should understand that chronic infection such as Lyme, CMV, and EBV are associated with chronic pain, and may pose a diagnostic challenge.

COVID-19 and Temporomandibular Disorder

The COVID-19 infection has changed the world forever. The effect COVID-19 has on the world of pain and orofacial pain, in general, and TMD pain, in particular, may not be any different. The effects of COVID-19 infection on TMD-associated pain are due to multifactorial reasons, including, but not limited to, the stress, anxiety, isolation, immune effects, and effects of the virus on the various tissues and systems.[66,67] In addition, there is mounting evidence of the effect of cortisol on the frequency and severity of SRB, which in turn, may be comorbid with TMD.[68] Respiratory viruses including COVID-19 have been shown to induce autoimmune responses, vasculitis, arthritis, and demyelinating conditions.[69] The clinical/immunologic signs and symptoms of post–COVID-19 syndrome, many a times, mimic RA and SLE.[70] The role of infectious agents such as COVID-19 in inducing autoimmunity and its subsequent effects on joints, muscles, and tissues is only being elucidated in the current literature.[71–73] Conceivably, the same or similar effects with tissue destruction and chronic pain are also possible in the TMJ, associated structures, and the masticatory musculature. Further, significant afflictions of the musculoskeletal system, acute, chronic, and long term, have been reported with patients with COVID-19.[70] The most recent literature describes mechanism of how COVID-19 virus disrupts muscle homeostasis and cause myalgia, muscle injury, and myopathy.[74] The clinician attempting to manage TMD and TMD pain should familiarize with the current literature, and anticipate complexities associated with COVID-19 infection.

Endocrinological Disorders

Several endocrinologic disorders have been shown to have association with TMD and TMD pain.[75] However, some hormonal association has been shown to be hypoalgesic with regards to TMD pain.[76–78] Estrogens, in general, have been identified as proalgesic in terms of general body pain as well as TMD pain.[79] Hormonal influences in maintaining TMD pain have been shown in studies related to oral contraceptive medications.[80] Progesterones have been shown to be hypoalgesic in relation to TMD pain.[81] There is increasing evidence of higher pain and severity of TMD in patients with polycystic ovarian syndrome.[82,83] Fatigability, myalgia, and associated higher TMD prevalence were found in patients with thyroid disorders.[75,84] It has been proposed that approximately 10% of patients with myofascial pain (including TMD-associated myofascial pain) have hypothyroidism.[85] Myalgia is a prominent feature in autoimmune thyroiditis.[86] Studies have revealed significant muscle fatigability in hypothyroid mice.[87] The role of thyroid hormones in preventing sarcopenia and myopathies has also been shown.[88] The clinician should be aware of the potential robust interaction between endocrinological disorders and TMD pain.

Drug-Induced Myalgia

Several drugs have been shown to cause, induce, and aggravate localized/global myalgia. These include, but not limited to, statins,[89–92] antimetabolites,[93] proton pump inhibitors,[94] and bisphosphonates.[95–97] The clinician dealing with TMD-associated pain should take a proper history to find out the possibility of a temporal relationship of the start or adjustment of dosage of any such medications to the onset of, and change in pain patterns. The known classes of drugs that induce myopathies and myalgias are given in **Table 2**.

Joint Hypermobility and Associated Syndromes

Joint hypermobility syndrome (JHS) was initially defined as the occurrence of musculoskeletal symptoms in the presence of joint laxity and hypermobility in otherwise healthy individuals. It is important to differentiate between the terms joint hypermobility (JH) and JHS. JH is defined as an excessive range of motion of a joint taking into consideration the patient's gender, age, and ethnic background. Usually this range is greater in women, younger people, and those of Asian or African origin.[101,102] By definition, JH only becomes JHS when symptoms attributable to JH occur. The

Table 2
Drugs associated with myopathy and/or myalgia[98–100]

Class	Examples	Class	Examples
Statins	Rosuvastatin Atorvastatin Simvastatin Fluvastatin	Antiviral	Zidovudine Ritonavir Lamivudine Stavudine
Antimetabolites	Doxorubicin Cisplatin 5-Fluorouracil cystemustine Cyclophosphamide	Antitubercular agents	Rifampicin Ethambutol Pyrazinamide
Proton Pump Inhibitors	Omeprazole Pantoprazole Lansoprazole Esomeprazole Abeprazole	Antibiotics	Nalidixic acid Ciprofloxacin Enoxacin Levofloxacin Metronidazole
Bisphosphonates	Alendronate Ibandronate Pamidronate Risedronate Zoledronate	Antifungal	Amphotericin B Terbinafine
Steroids		Antithyroid	Carbimazole Propylthiouracil
Cardio vascular agents	Captopril Enalapril Methyldopa Bumetanide	Calcium channel blockers	Nifedipine

likely scenario is that most hypermobile subjects experience little or no such symptoms.[103,104]

In other individuals, symptoms may develop during childhood, adolescence, or adult life, depending on lifestyle and exposure to injury.[102] The diagnostic criteria most commonly used today and still considered the yardstick for proposed hypermobility scales is the Beighton scale.[105,106] It must be noted that the Beighton's scale considers the range of motion at multiple established joints. The comorbidities that commonly occur with JHS are presented in **Fig. 1**.

When generalized JH is accompanied by pain in 4 joints or greater during a period 3 months or greater in the absence of other conditions that cause chronic pain, the hypermobility syndrome or JHS may be diagnosed.[107] In addition, generalized joint hypermobility (GJH) is also a clinical sign that is frequently present in hereditary diseases of the connective tissue (HDCT), such as the Marfan syndrome, osteogenesis imperfecta, the Ehler–Danlos syndrome, and the Stickler syndrome. Overlap occurs between JHS and HDCT.[107]

Some decades ago, JHS was considered as a benign condition but now it is recognized as a significant contributor to chronic musculoskeletal pain, besides its impact on other organs.[108,109] Patients with JHS often have diffuse, chronic complaints that are inconsistent with pain originating from the musculoskeletal system. It has been estimated that among individuals with GJH, approximately 3.3% of women, and 0.6% of men develop chronic complaints.[110] Among EDS patients, chronic widespread pain is quite common. Incidence of chronic pain has been reported as high as 90% in EDS patients.[111] Some studies showed a higher prevalence of pain in hypermobile than in classic EDS.[102,112]

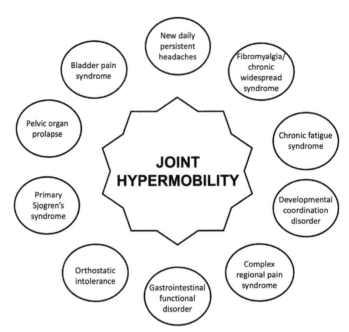

Fig. 1. Comorbidities associated with joint hypermobility syndrome.

The specific underlying causes and mechanisms of pain in JHS and EDS remain poorly understood. Different factors likely contributing to the generation and chronicity of pain include nociceptive pain, directly based on structural changes in affected joints, muscle, and connective tissue; neuropathic pain; impaired proprioception and muscle weakness; and central sensitization.[113] The comorbidities/coexisting conditions presenting with JHS may include reduced proprioception, premature OA, soft tissue pain, psychological disorders, and chronic pain.[114] Central sensitization syndromes such as fibromyalgia are also associated with JHS.[115]

Sleep

Sleep and pain are currently believed to have a bidirectional relationship, with impairment of sleep affecting the experience of pain, and the latter affecting sleep quality. Impairment of sleep is considered a strong predictor of pain.[116] Sleep disorders such as insomnia, obstructive sleep apnea, sleep-related breathing disorders, and sleep-related movement disorders have shown to have association with pain.[117,118] The effect of sleep deprivation in increasing pain perception has been shown in multiple studies in humans and animals.[119–121] Painful TMD symptoms have shown to be more associated with disturbed sleep, and the intensity of the same was shown to be having negative association with sleep quality.[122] TMD and TMD-associated pain are highly associated with insomnia, especially in women.[123] Patients with TMD with associated disability were shown to have high plasma proinflammatory cytokine levels, and increased scores on Epworth Sleepiness Scale and Pittsburgh's Sleep Quality Index.[124] Sleep parameters may be important guides to help predicting the success of TMD pain management and may have a prognostic value. Improving sleep quality is crucial for an effective TMD pain management and for an overall improvement in QoL for patients with TMD.[67,125]

CLINICAL PEARLS

In a patient with myalgia (regional, diffuse, or global), the clinician may want to consider the myalgia protocol, which may include, but not limited to a complete blood count with differential, a complete metabolic panel with electrolytes, erythrocyte sedimentation rate, C-reactive protein, antinuclear antibodies, anemia panel, total iron-binding capacity with ferritin (especially when bruxism and restless leg syndrome coexist), vitamin D assay, and a thyroid panel. The decision to order any, some, or all of these parameters should come from the clinician's acumen and a thorough medical history and clinical examination. When patients with TMD present with bilateral jaw joint pain with concomitant dry mouth, masticatory myalgia, other arthralgias, and accompanied by other systemic manifestations, the possibility of RA and SLE should be explored. Patients, both adults and children, presenting with anterior open bite, possible retrognathia, and apparent tongue thrust, with associated systemic features are strong candidates to be worked up for RA. When a patient with TMD aged older than 60 years presents with generalized myalgia, unilateral or bilateral facial/head and neck pain, with a history of anemia or Raynaud's phenomenon, a rule out for polymyalgia rheumatica (PMR) and giant cell arteritis must be considered. For patients with TMD presenting with global pain, facial pain, sensitivity to cold, and feeling of tiredness/lethargy, a thyroid function test is highly recommended. In a patient presenting with TMD pain, and other orofacial pain complaints, the possible role of chronic infections such as Lyme, EBV, CMV, and COVID-19 should be considered and explored. The clinician managing TMD and TMD-associated pain must be aware and updated with the literature regarding the possibility of a myriad of TMD signs and symptoms that are probably hitherto either scantily described or not described at all in the literature. The clinician should carefully interview the patient with TMD regarding the temporal relationship between the TMD pain symptoms (or worsening thereof) and infection by COVID-19.

DISCLOSURE

D.C. Thomas, E. Eliav, A.R. Garcia, and M. Fatahzadeh have no commercial or financial conflicts of interest. No funding was received for this article.

REFERENCES

1. Health Nlo. First Evidence-Based Diagnostic Criteria Published for Temporomandibular Disorders (NIDCR)-2/3/14. 2014.

2. Valesan LF, Da-Cas CD, Réus JC, et al. Prevalence of temporomandibular joint disorders: a systematic review and meta-analysis. Clin Oral Investig 2021;25(2): 441–53.

3. List T, Jensen RH. Temporomandibular disorders: old ideas and new concepts. Cephalalgia 2017;37(7):692–704.

4. Zelaya CE, Dahlhamer JM, Lucas JW, et al. Chronic pain and high-impact chronic pain among US adults. NCHS Data Brief 2020;390:1–8.

5. Piga A. Impact of bone disease and pain in thalassemia. Hematology Am Soc Hematol Educ Program 2017;2017(1):272–7.

6. Caracas Mda S, Jales SP, Jales Neto LH, et al. Temporomandibular joint arthritis in sickle cell disease: a case report. Oral Surg Oral Med Oral Pathol Oral Radiol 2013;115(2):e31–5.

7. Mehra P, Wolford LM. Serum nutrient deficiencies in the patient with complex temporomandibular joint problems. Proc (Bayl Univ Med Cent) 2008;21(3): 243–7.
8. Kui A, Buduru S, Labunet A, et al. Vitamin D and Temporomandibular Disorders: What Do We Know So Far? Nutrients 2021;13(4). https://doi.org/10.3390/nu13041286.
9. Shen M, Luo Y, Niu Y, et al. 1,25(OH)2D deficiency induces temporomandibular joint osteoarthritis via secretion of senescence-associated inflammatory cytokines. Bone 2013;55(2):400–9.
10. Stohler CS. Muscle-related temporomandibular disorders. J Orofac Pain 1999; 13(4):273–84.
11. Winocur-Arias O, Friedman-Rubin P, Abu Ras K, et al. Local myalgia compared to myofascial pain with referral according to the DC/TMD: Axis I and II results. BMC Oral Health 2022;22(1):27.
12. Thomas DC, Kohli D, Chen N, et al. Orofacial manifestations of rheumatoid arthritis and systemic lupus erythematosus: a narrative review. Quintessence Int 2021;52(5):454–66.
13. Abramoff B, Caldera FE. Osteoarthritis: pathology, diagnosis, and treatment options. Med Clin North Am 2020;104(2):293–311.
14. Daily JW, Yang M, Park S. Efficacy of turmeric extracts and curcumin for alleviating the symptoms of joint arthritis: a systematic review and meta-analysis of randomized clinical trials. J Med Food 2016;19(8):717–29.
15. Bessa-Nogueira RV, Vasconcelos BC, Duarte AP, et al. Targeted assessment of the temporomandibular joint in patients with rheumatoid arthritis. J Oral Maxillofac Surg 2008;66(9):1804–11.
16. Badel T, Savić Pavičin I, Krapac L, et al. Psoriatic arthritis and temporomandibular joint involvement - literature review with a reported case. Acta Dermatovenerol Croat 2014;22(2):114–21.
17. Roopa R, Malarkodi T, Azariah E, Warrier AS. The involvement of temporomandibular joint in psoriatic arthritis: a report of a rare case. Cureus 2021;13(12): e20392.
18. Falisi G, Gatto R, Di Paolo C, et al. A female psoriatic arthritis patient involving the TMJ. Case Rep Dent 2021;2021:6638638.
19. Franks AS. Temporomandibular joint arthrosis associated with psoriasis. report of a case. Oral Surg Oral Med Oral Pathol 1965;19:301–3.
20. Yamamoto T. Psoriatic arthritis: from a dermatological perspective. Eur J Dermatol 2011;21(5):660–6.
21. Alinaghi F, Calov M, Kristensen LE, et al. Prevalence of psoriatic arthritis in patients with psoriasis: A systematic review and meta-analysis of observational and clinical studies. J Am Acad Dermatol 2019;80(1):251–65.e19.
22. Mease PJ, Gladman DD, Papp KA, et al. Prevalence of rheumatologist-diagnosed psoriatic arthritis in patients with psoriasis in European/North American dermatology clinics. J Am Acad Dermatol 2013;69(5):729–35.
23. Okkesim A, Adisen MZ, Misirlioglu M. Temporomandibular joint involvement in psoriatic arthritis. Niger J Clin Pract 2017;20(11):1501–4.
24. Chandran V, Raychaudhuri SP. Geoepidemiology and environmental factors of psoriasis and psoriatic arthritis. J Autoimmun 2010;34(3):J314–21.
25. Nograles KE, Brasington RD, Bowcock AM. New insights into the pathogenesis and genetics of psoriatic arthritis. Nat Clin Pract Rheumatol 2009;5(2):83–91.

26. Kulkarni AU, Gadre PK, Kulkarni PA, et al. Diagnosing psoriatic arthritis of the temporomandibular joint: a study in radiographic images. BMJ Case Rep 2013;2013:2013–010301.
27. Könönen M, Wolf J, Kilpinen E, et al. Radiographic signs in the temporomandibular and hand joints in patients with psoriatic arthritis. Acta Odontol Scand 1991; 49(4):191–6.
28. Covert L, Mater HV, Hechler BL. Comprehensive Management of Rheumatic Diseases Affecting the Temporomandibular Joint. Diagnostics (Basel) 2021; 11(3). https://doi.org/10.3390/diagnostics11030409.
29. Tiwari V, Brent LH. Psoriatic Arthritis. StatPearls. StatPearls Publishing Copyright © 2022, 2022 Copyright © 2022, StatPearls Publishing LLC.; 2022.
30. O'Connor RC, Fawthrop F, Salha R, et al. Management of the temporomandibular joint in inflammatory arthritis: Involvement of surgical procedures. Eur J Rheumatol 2017;4(2):151–6.
31. Crincoli V, Di Comite M, Di Bisceglie MB, et al. Temporomandibular Disorders in Psoriasis Patients with and without Psoriatic Arthritis: An Observational Study. Int J Med Sci 2015;12(4):341–8.
32. Könönen M. Craniomandibular disorders in psoriatic arthritis. Correlations between subjective symptoms, clinical signs, and radiographic changes. Acta Odontol Scand 1986;44(6):369–75.
33. Popat R, Matthews N, Connor S. Psoriatic arthritis of the temporomandibular joint–a surgical alternative to treating a medical problem. Oral Surg 2010; 3(1–2):47–50.
34. Melchiorre D, Calderazzi A, Maddali Bongi S, et al. A comparison of ultrasonography and magnetic resonance imaging in the evaluation of temporomandibular joint involvement in rheumatoid arthritis and psoriatic arthritis. Rheumatology (Oxford) 2003;42(5):673–6.
35. Sarzi-Puttini P, Batticciotto A, Atzeni F, et al. Medical cannabis and cannabinoids in rheumatology: where are we now? Expert Rev Clin Immunol 2019;15(10): 1019–32.
36. Masala IF, Caso F, Sarzi-Puttini P, et al. Acute and chronic pain in orthopaedic and rheumatologic diseases: mechanisms and characteristics. Clin Exp Rheumatol 2017;105(3):127–31.
37. Firestein & Kelley's textbook of rheumatology. 11th edition, 2021.
38. Tani C, Carli L, Stagnaro C, et al. Imaging of joints in systemic lupus erythematosus. Clin Exp Rheumatol 2018;36:S68–73.
39. Bhattacharyya I, Chehal H, Gremillion H, et al. Gout of the temporomandibular joint: a review of the literature. J Am Dent Assoc 2010;141(8):979–85.
40. Henry CH, Whittum-Hudson JA, Tull GT, et al. Reactive arthritis and internal derangement of the temporomandibular joint. Oral Surg Oral Med Oral Pathol Oral Radiol Endod 2007;104(1):e22–6.
41. Di Franco M, Guzzo MP, Spinelli FR, et al. Pain and systemic lupus erythematosus. Rev Reumatismo 2014;66(1):33–8.
42. Crincoli V, Piancino MG, Iannone F, et al. in Systemic Lupus Erythematosus Patients: An Observational Study of Symptoms and Signs. Int J Med Sci 2020; 17(2):153–60.
43. Staniszewski K, Lygre H, Berge T, et al. Serum Analysis in Patients with Temporomandibular Disorders: A Controlled Cross-Sectional Study in Norway. Pain Res Manag 2019;2019:1360725.

44. Madani A, Shamsian SA, Layegh P, et al. Are certain factors involved in calcium metabolism associated with temporomandibular disorders? Cranio 2021;39(3): 202–8.
45. Wu Z, Malihi Z, Stewart AW, et al. Effect of Vitamin D Supplementation on Pain: A Systematic Review and Meta-analysis. Pain Physician 2016;19(7):415–27.
46. Yong WC, Sanguankeo A, Upala S. Effect of vitamin D supplementation in chronic widespread pain: a systematic review and meta-analysis. Clin Rheumatol 2017;36(12):2825–33.
47. de Oliveira DL, Hirotsu C, Tufik S, et al. The interfaces between vitamin D, sleep and pain. J Endocrinol 2017;234(1):R23–36.
48. Alkhatatbeh MJ, Hmoud ZL, Abdul-Razzak KK, et al. Self-reported sleep bruxism is associated with vitamin D deficiency and low dietary calcium intake: a case-control study. BMC Oral Health 2021;21(1):21.
49. Elma Ö, Yilmaz ST, Deliens T, et al. Chronic Musculoskeletal Pain and Nutrition: Where Are We and Where Are We Heading? PM R 2020;12(12):1268–78.
50. Petrov ME, Howard G, Grandner MA, et al. Sleep duration and risk of incident stroke by age, sex, and race: the regards study. Neurology 2018;91(18): e1702–9.
51. Koedel U, Fingerle V, Pfister HW. Lyme neuroborreliosis-epidemiology, diagnosis and management. Nat Rev Neurol 2015;11(8):446–56.
52. Hydén D, Roberg M, Forsberg P, et al. Acute "idiopathic" peripheral facial palsy: clinical, serological, and cerebrospinal fluid findings and effects of corticosteroids. Am J Otolaryngol 1993;14(3):179–86.
53. Osiewicz M, Manfredini D, Biesiada G, et al. Differences between palpation and static/dynamic tests to diagnose painful temporomandibular disorders in patients with Lyme disease. Clin Oral Investig 2019;23(12):4411–6.
54. Osiewicz M, Manfredini D, Biesiada G, et al. Prevalence of function-dependent temporomandibular joint and masticatory muscle pain, and predictors of temporomandibular disorders among patients with lyme disease. J Clin Med 2019; 8(7). https://doi.org/10.3390/jcm8070929.
55. Rebman AW, Aucott JN. Post-treatment lyme disease as a model for persistent symptoms in lyme disease. Front Med (Lausanne) 2020;7:57.
56. Shadick NA, Phillips CB, Sangha O, et al. Musculoskeletal and neurologic outcomes in patients with previously treated Lyme disease. Ann Intern Med 1999; 131(12):919–26.
57. Manicklal S, Emery VC, Lazzarotto T, et al. The "silent" global burden of congenital cytomegalovirus. Clin Microbiol Rev 2013;26(1):86–102.
58. Staras SA, Dollard SC, Radford KW, et al. Seroprevalence of cytomegalovirus infection in the United States, 1988-1994. Clin Infect Dis 2006;43(9):1143–51.
59. Nolan N, Halai UA, Regunath H, et al. Primary cytomegalovirus infection in immunocompetent adults in the United States - a case series. IDCases 2017; 10:123–6.
60. Yamani N, Olesen J. New daily persistent headache: a systematic review on an enigmatic disorder. J Headache Pain 2019;20(1):80.
61. Meineri P, Torre E, Rota E, et al. New daily persistent headache: clinical and serological characteristics in a retrospective study. Neurol Sci 2004;3:S281–2.
62. Drosu NC, Edelman ER, Housman DE. Tenofovir prodrugs potently inhibit Epstein-Barr virus lytic DNA replication by targeting the viral DNA polymerase. Proc Natl Acad Sci U S A 2020;117(22):12368–74.
63. Ascherio A, Munger KL. EBV and Autoimmunity. Curr Top Microbiol Immunol 2015;390(Pt 1):365–85.

64. Diaz-Mitoma F, Vanast WJ, Tyrrell DL. Increased frequency of Epstein-Barr virus excretion in patients with new daily persistent headaches. Lancet 1987;1(8530): 411–5.

65. Feced Olmos CM, Fernández Matilla M, Robustillo Villarino M, et al. Joint involvement secondary to Epstein-Barr virus. Reumatol Clin 2016;12(2):100–2.

66. Colonna A, Guarda-Nardini L, Ferrari M, et al. COVID-19 pandemic and the psyche, bruxism, temporomandibular disorders triangle. Cranio 2021;15:1–6.

67. Peixoto KO, Resende C, Almeida EO, et al. Association of sleep quality and psychological aspects with reports of bruxism and TMD in Brazilian dentists during the COVID-19 pandemic. J Appl Oral Sci 2021;29:e20201089.

68. Saccomanno S, Bernabei M, Scoppa F, et al. Coronavirus lockdown as a major life stressor: does it affect TMD symptoms? Int J Environ Res Public Health 2020; 17(23). https://doi.org/10.3390/ijerph17238907.

69. Novelli L, Motta F, De Santis M, et al. The JANUS of chronic inflammatory and autoimmune diseases onset during COVID-19-A systematic review of the literature. J Autoimmun 2021;117:102592.

70. Larionova R, Byvaltsev K, Kravtsova O, et al. SARS-Cov2 acute and post-active infection in the context of autoimmune and chronic inflammatory diseases. J Transl Autoimmun 2022;5:100154.

71. Latorre D. Autoimmunity and SARS-CoV-2 infection: unraveling the link in neurological disorders. Eur J Immunol 2022. https://doi.org/10.1002/eji.202149475.

72. Martone AM, Tosato M, Ciciarello F, et al. Sarcopenia as potential biological substrate of long COVID-19 syndrome: prevalence, clinical features, and risk factors. J Cachexia Sarcopenia Muscle 2022. https://doi.org/10.1002/jcsm.12931.

73. Pires RE, Reis IGN, Waldolato GS, et al. What do we need to know about musculoskeletal manifestations of COVID-19?: a systematic review. JBJS Rev 2022; 10(6). https://doi.org/10.2106/JBJS.RVW.22.00013.

74. Galea M, Agius M, Vassallo N. Neurological manifestations and pathogenic mechanisms of COVID-19. Neurol Res 2022;44(7):571–82.

75. Grozdinska A, Hofmann E, Schmid M, et al. Prevalence of temporomandibular disorders in patients with Hashimoto thyroiditis. J Orofac Orthop 2018;79(4): 277–88.

76. Li YX, Li JH, Guo Y, et al. Oxytocin inhibits hindpaw hyperalgesia induced by orofacial inflammation combined with stress. Mol Pain 2022;18. 17448069221089591.

77. Javed F, Ahmed HB, Zafar MS, et al. Testosterone decreases temporomandibular joint nociception"- A systematic review of studies on animal models. Arch Oral Biol 2022;139:105430.

78. Fischer L, Clemente JT, Tambeli CH. The protective role of testosterone in the development of temporomandibular joint pain. J Pain 2007;8(5):437–42.

79. Jedynak B, Jaworska-Zaremba M, Grzechocińska B, et al. TMD in females with menstrual disorders. Int J Environ Res Public Health 2021;18(14). https://doi.org/10.3390/ijerph18147263.

80. Gaynor SM, Fillingim RB, Zolnoun DA, et al. Association of hormonal contraceptive use with headache and temporomandibular pain: the oppera study. J Oral Facial Pain Headache 2021;35(2):105–12.

81. Bi RY, Zhang XY, Zhang P, et al. Progesterone attenuates allodynia of inflamed temporomandibular joint through modulating voltage-gated sodium channel 1.7 in trigeminal ganglion. Pain Res Manag 2020;2020:6582586.

82. Soydan SS, Deniz K, Uckan S, et al. Is the incidence of temporomandibular disorder increased in polycystic ovary syndrome? Br J Oral Maxillofac Surg 2014; 52(9):822–6.

83. Yazici H, Taskin MI, Guney G, et al. The novel relationship between polycystic ovary syndrome and temporomandibular joint disorders. J Stomatol Oral Maxillofac Surg 2021;122(6):544–8.

84. Jordan B, Uer O, Buchholz T, et al. Physical fatigability and muscle pain in patients with Hashimoto thyroiditis. J Neurol 2021;268(7):2441–9.

85. Gerwin RD. A review of myofascial pain and fibromyalgia–factors that promote their persistence. Acupunct Med 2005;23(3):121–34.

86. Punzi L, Betterle C. Chronic autoimmune thyroiditis and rheumatic manifestations. Joint Bone Spine 2004;71(4):275–83.

87. Elnakish MT, Schultz EJ, Gearinger RL, et al. Differential involvement of various sources of reactive oxygen species in thyroxin-induced hemodynamic changes and contractile dysfunction of the heart and diaphragm muscles. Free Radic Biol Med 2015;83:252–61.

88. Bloise FF, Oliveira TS, Cordeiro A, et al. Thyroid hormones play role in sarcopenia and myopathies. Front Physiol 2018;9:560.

89. Patel PP, Jackson CD. When statins get physical: a curious cause of statin myopathy. South Med J 2022;115(4):266–9.

90. Mammen AL. Statin-associated myalgias and muscle injury-recognizing and managing both while still lowering the low-density lipoprotein. Rheum Dis Clin North Am 2022;48(2):445–54.

91. Pergolizzi JV Jr, Coluzzi F, Colucci RD, et al. Statins and muscle pain. Expert Rev Clin Pharmacol 2020;13(3):299–310.

92. Thompson PD, Panza G, Zaleski A, et al. Statin-associated side effects. J Am Coll Cardiol 2016;67(20):2395–410.

93. Fitzgerald K, White S, Borodovsky A, et al. A highly durable rnai therapeutic inhibitor of PCSK9. N Engl J Med 2017;376(1):41–51.

94. Grossner T, Haberkorn U, Gotterbarm T. Evaluation of the impact of different pain medication and proton pump inhibitors on the osteogenic differentiation potential of hMSCs using (99m)Tc-HDP labelling. Life (Basel) 2021;11(4). https://doi.org/10.3390/life11040339.

95. Lim SY, Bolster MB. What can we do about musculoskeletal pain from bisphosphonates? Cleve Clin J Med 2018;85(9):675–8.

96. Tsimicalis A, Boitor M, Ferland CE, et al. Pain and quality of life of children and adolescents with osteogenesis imperfecta over a bisphosphonate treatment cycle. Eur J Pediatr 2018;177(6):891–902.

97. Papapetrou PD. Bisphosphonate-associated adverse events. Hormones (Athens) 2009;8(2):96–110.

98. Bannwarth B. Drug-induced myopathies. Expert Opin Drug Saf 2002;1(1): 65–70.

99. Holder K. Myalgias and myopathies: drug-induced myalgias and myopathies. FP essentials 2016;440:23–7.

100. Dalakas MC. Toxic and drug-induced myopathies. J Neurol Neurosurg Psychiatry 2009;80(8):832–8.

101. Carbonell-Bobadilla N, Rodríguez-Álvarez AA, Rojas-García G, et al. [Joint hypermobility syndrome]. Acta Ortop Mex 2020;34(6):441–9.

102. Engelbert RH, Juul-Kristensen B, Pacey V, et al. The evidence-based rationale for physical therapy treatment of children, adolescents, and adults diagnosed

with joint hypermobility syndrome/hypermobile Ehlers Danlos syndrome. Am J Med Genet C Semin Med Genet 2017;175(1):158–67.

103. Tinkle BT. Symptomatic joint hypermobility. Best Pract Res Clin Rheumatol 2020; 34(3):101508.

104. Tinkle BT, Levy HP. Symptomatic joint hypermobility: the hypermobile type of ehlers-danlos syndrome and the hypermobility spectrum disorders. Med Clin North Am 2019;103(6):1021–33.

105. Stendal Robinson H, Lindgren A, Bjelland EK. Generalized joint hypermobility and risk of pelvic girdle pain in pregnancy: does body mass index matter? Physiother Theor Pract 2021;14:1–8.

106. Steinberg N, Hershkovitz I, Zeev A, et al. Joint hypermobility and joint range of motion in young dancers. J Clin Rheumatol 2016;22(4):171–8.

107. Hakim AJ, Grahame R. Non-musculoskeletal symptoms in joint hypermobility syndrome. Indirect evidence for autonomic dysfunction? Rheumatology (Oxford) 2004;43(9):1194–5.

108. T VANM Huijnen IP, Engelbert RH, Verbunt JA. Are chronic musculoskeletal pain and generalized joint hypermobility disabling contributors to physical functioning? Eur J Phys Rehabil Med 2021;57(5):747–57.

109. Reuter PR, Fichthorn KR. Prevalence of generalized joint hypermobility, musculoskeletal injuries, and chronic musculoskeletal pain among American university students. PeerJ 2019;7:e7625.

110. Scheper MC, de Vries JE, Verbunt J, et al. Chronic pain in hypermobility syndrome and Ehlers-Danlos syndrome (hypermobility type): it is a challenge. J Pain Res 2015;8:591–601.

111. Sacheti A, Szemere J, Bernstein B, et al. Chronic pain is a manifestation of the Ehlers-Danlos syndrome. J Pain Symptom Manage 1997;14(2):88–93.

112. Tinkle B, Castori M, Berglund B, et al. Hypermobile Ehlers-Danlos syndrome (a.k.a. Ehlers-Danlos syndrome Type III and Ehlers-Danlos syndrome hypermobility type): clinical description and natural history. Am J Med Genet C Semin Med Genet 2017;175(1):48–69.

113. Syx D, De Wandele I, Rombaut L, et al. Hypermobility, the Ehlers-Danlos syndromes and chronic pain. Clin Exp Rheumatol 2017;107(5):116–22.

114. Hall MG, Ferrell WR, Sturrock RD, et al. The effect of the hypermobility syndrome on knee joint proprioception. Br J Rheumatol 1995;34(2):121–5.

115. Sahin N, Atik A, Dogan E. Clinical and demographic characteristics and functional status of the patients with fibromyalgia syndrome. North Clin Istanb 2014;1(2):89–94.

116. Finan PH, Goodin BR, Smith MT. The association of sleep and pain: an update and a path forward. J Pain 2013;14(12):1539–52.

117. Athar W, Card ME, Charokopos A, et al. Obstructive sleep apnea and pain intensity in young adults. Ann Am Thorac Soc 2020;17(10):1273–8.

118. Lam KK, Kunder S, Wong J, et al. Obstructive sleep apnea, pain, and opioids: is the riddle solved? Curr Opin Anaesthesiol 2016;29(1):134–40.

119. Roehrs T, Hyde M, Blaisdell B, et al. Sleep loss and REM sleep loss are hyperalgesic. Sleep 2006;29(2):145–51.

120. Kundermann B, Krieg JC, Schreiber W, et al. The effect of sleep deprivation on pain. Pain Res Manag 2004;9(1):25–32.

121. Onen SH, Alloui A, Gross A, et al. The effects of total sleep deprivation, selective sleep interruption and sleep recovery on pain tolerance thresholds in healthy subjects. J Sleep Res 2001;10(1):35–42.

122. Fernandes G, van Selms MKA, Lobbezoo F, et al. Subjective sleep complaints were associated with painful temporomandibular disorders in adolescents: The Epidor-Adolescere study. J Oral Rehabil 2022;49(9):849–59.
123. Lerman SF, Mun CJ, Hunt CA, et al. Insomnia with objective short sleep duration in women with temporomandibular joint disorder: quantitative sensory testing, inflammation and clinical pain profiles. Sleep Med 2022;90:26–35.
124. Park JW, Chung JW. Inflammatory cytokines and sleep disturbance in patients with temporomandibular disorders. J Oral Facial Pain Headache 2016;30(1):27–33.
125. Bergmann A, Edelhoff D, Schubert O, et al. Effect of treatment with a full-occlusion biofeedback splint on sleep bruxism and TMD pain: a randomized controlled clinical trial. Clin Oral Investig 2020;24(11):4005–18.

Temporomandibular Disorders and Dental Occlusion: What Do We Know so Far?

Davis C. Thomas, BDS, DDS, MSD, MSc Med, MSc[a,b,*],
Steven R. Singer, DDS[a], Stanley Markman, DDS[a]

KEYWORDS

- Temporomandibular disorders ● Occlusion ● Orofacial pain ● TMD
- Occlusal disharmonies ● Malocclusion

KEY POINTS

- Occlusion, occlusal factors, and occlusal disharmonies seem to have no causal relationship with temporomandibular disorders (TMDs).
- Correction of occlusal disharmonies do not prevent TMDs from occurring nor treat it.
- Not correcting malocclusion and occlusal disharmonies does not cause TMD.
- Succinct knowledge about cause and pathogenesis of TMDs is of paramount importance to the dental clinician.
- Aggressive and irreversible dental treatment with a view to treat TMDs is not warranted or supported by current sound scientific literature.

INTRODUCTION

Over the last several decades, the science of dentistry has evolved exponentially. One of the most heated debates in dentistry has been what occlusion or occlusal scheme is ideal for optimum function, in addition to the hope of preventing and ameliorating temporomandibular disorders (TMDs). Fundamental question that has almost never been fully answered and elucidated has been "Is there a causal relationship between occlusal disharmonies/malocclusion and TMDs?" Various subspecialties of dentistry have attempted to define ideal occlusion with a resultant slightly different viewpoints to vastly varying philosophies. Literature published to date does not seem to support one scheme of occlusion over another, in the context of preventing or ameliorating TMDs; this has led to considerable confusion in dentistry,

[a] Department of Diagnostic Sciences, Rutgers School of Dental Medicine, 110 Bergen Street, Newark, NJ 07103, USA; [b] Eastman Institute of Oral Health, Rochester, NY 14642, USA
* Corresponding author. Department of Diagnostic Sciences, Rutgers School of Dental Medicine, 110 Bergen Street, PO Box 1709, Newark, NJ 07101-1709.
E-mail address: davisct1@gmail.com

Dent Clin N Am 67 (2023) 299–308
https://doi.org/10.1016/j.cden.2022.11.002
0011-8532/23/© 2022 Elsevier Inc. All rights reserved.

with a plethora of widely ranging hypotheses and postulations, in an attempt to define the "ideal occlusion." Further, one of the most long-standing questions in dentistry has been whether a person who naturally developed a malocclusion is predisposed to the occurrence of TMDs. The same apparent confusion also led to a myriad of suggestions and "guidelines" under the principles of the various specialties of dentistry. The magnitude and complexity of this issue was such that dental students over the last several decades jovially opined that ideal occlusion depends on the department you land in. The most recent literature over the last few decades seem to indicate that occlusal disharmonies and malocclusions do not predispose to or cause TMDs. Further, correction of these occlusal disharmonies and malocclusions does not result in predictable relief of TMD symptoms. It is paramount that an astute clinician should be able to screen for TMDs, manage, and ensure prompt appropriate referrals to a specialist. Aggressive management modalities that involve extensive, irreversible dental treatments in an attempt to either prevent, ameliorate, or treat TMDs should be avoided.

The prevalence of TMDs is generally estimated between 5% and 12% in the general population.[1,2] Among the causes for nondental chronic orofacial pain, TMDs are considered the most common.[3] One of the fundamental issues for the extensive variations in the way that TMDs were interpreted in various philosophies is the confusion in defining what constitutes a TMD. Temporomandibular joint (TMJ) disc displacement with reduction is considered the most common TMD entity.[1,4,5] There have been various hypotheses in the last several decades of dental literature in an attempt to explain what exactly causes a TMJ disc displacement. There has not been a clear consensus in this regard either. In this article, the authors have attempted to explore, based on literature, whether there is a causality between malocclusion (developmental/natural or iatrogenic) and TMD.

OCCLUSAL CHANGES AS A SEQUELA OF TEMPOROMANDIBULAR DISORDER

As opposed to the concept of occlusal disharmonies and malocclusion "causing" TMDs, the more appropriate philosophy seems to be TMDs causing occlusal changes.[6] Both changes in the masticatory muscles and in the TMJs have the potential to cause occlusal changes. These changes may include, but not limited to, anterior/posterior open bite, uneven occlusal contacts, crossbites, abnormal occlusal curves, and other abnormalities in occlusal patterns.[6-11] Both acute and chronic TMDs may cause occlusal changes. The acute entities may include myospasm, muscle weakness, and capsulitis of the joint. Chronic TMD conditions that cause changes in the occlusion include, but not limited to, changes secondary to arthritides, chronic TMJ inflammatory conditions, systemic conditions that affect the joints, and other local and systemic entities.[12,13] Conditions such as myospasm, if left untreated, has the potential to cause contracture and may lead to occlusal changes. Idiopathic condylar resorption is a poorly understood cause of anterior open bite, which sometimes may be progressive. TMD and TMD-related pain show no anticipated relationship with either occlusal or postural abnormalities.[14] Changes in static or dynamic occlusal factors have not shown to be causally related to TMDs.[15] Another small study of less than 50 subjects had proposed that excessive overjet was associated with an increase in risk of TMD.[16] However, the same study also reported that the predictive value of these variables was minimal with regard to estimating the individual's risk for TMD. A 2007 systematic review of the literature looked at malocclusions, orthodontic treatment, and TMD symptoms and signs and found no association between malocclusions and significant signs and symptoms of TMD.[17]

OCCLUSION-TEMPOROMANDIBULAR DISORDER RELATIONSHIP: LONE-STANDING ARTICLES

There is at least one study referring to the role of "tightly locked occlusion" and TMD symptoms. In this isolated article,[18] the investigators had described special occlusal contacts delivering hypothesized angled occlusal forces on teeth, thereby bringing about TMD symptoms. However, further studies were not found on this principle. There have also been older articles that refer to the possible role of molar relationship, lateral guidance, and nonworking side contacts, to TMD symptomatology, but no such relationship was found.[19] Another recent study found a relatively high prevalence of TMD signs in patients with Parkinson disease with concomitant higher frequency of occlusal asymmetry. This finding, however, could not be independently verified.[20] Other electromyogram (EMG) studies apparently showed a higher masseter/temporalis muscle activity in patients with moderate-to-severe TMDs.[21] However, this study could not find any statistically significant difference in the occlusal contact patterns between patients with and without TMD. A plethora of isolated articles can be found in the literature attempting to link malocclusion, TMD, and several other variables; however, strong further studies are essential to come even close to a conclusion.

DEEP BITE/CROSSBITE: IS THERE A RELATIONSHIP WITH TEMPOROMANDIBULAR DISORDER?

In the very early TMD literature, malocclusions including deep bite, crossbite, and class II malocclusion among others were proposed to be causally related to TMDs. The current school of thought based on sound evidence is that such malocclusions do not predispose to and are not causally related to TMDs.[22] The conventional belief of static dental occlusal relationships such as deep bite, crossbite, eccentric contacts, and so on are associated with TMDs and are not supported by scientific data.[23,24] Any such relationship reported has been largely anecdotal. Some articles have proposed the role of crossbite in TMDs.[25–28] Recent studies have shown that when TMD coexist with bruxism, the concomitant presence of crossbite or deep bite is not a risk factor for pain or disc displacement.[29] Further, deep bite has shown to be not related to TMD pain or disc displacement.[30] Both anterior and posterior crossbites have been proposed to have no effect on disc displacement and some effect on TMD pain; however, no mechanism has been explained for this association.[30] To date, no conclusionary evidence exist in the published literature causally linking deep bite/crossbite to TMD or TMD pain. Correcting deep bite or crossbite with the sole purpose of preventing or managing TMD is therefore unwarranted.

OCCLUSAL INTERFERENCES AND TEMPOROMANDIBULAR DISORDER

The Glossary of Prosthodontic Terms (9th edition) defines occlusal interference as "any tooth contact that inhibits the remaining occluding surfaces from achieving stable and harmonious contacts" and "any undesirable occlusal contact."[31] Occlusal interferences in static and dynamic maxillomandibular relationships have long been thought to be causally related to TMDs. An attempt was made in 2009 by Cao and colleagues,[32] in trying to relate occlusal interferences experimentally induced to long-term hyperalgesia in the masticatory muscles in rats. This experiment seemed to indicate that hyperalgesia was induced in the masticatory muscles as a result of occlusal interferences. However, this was followed by Bereiter and colleagues in 2010 pointing out several "flaws" in the study design and conceptual errors in the 2009 pain article. Occlusal interferences failed to show any predictive or causal relationship to TMD pain.[17,33–35] A publication in late 1990s that looked at and summarized more than 20 combined human and animal studies published over a period of more than 60 years summarized that there is absolutely no proof that occlusal interferences cause TMD or TMD-associated pain.[33] A 2004 article also had concluded that occlusal features including interferences have negligible value in predicting TMD or TMD-related pain.[34] In light of mounting evidence in the literature of nonassociation of occlusal interferences and TMD, there is no current valid justification for eliminating or "adjusting" occlusal interferences with a sole purpose of managing or treating TMDs.

DEVELOPMENTAL MALOCCLUSION, FUNCTIONAL OCCLUSION, AND TEMPOROMANDIBULAR DISORDER

Occlusal abnormalities in the developing dentition, such as Class II malocclusion, deep bite, anterior crossbite, and so forth, are traditionally believed to be either causing TMD or associated with TMD.[36] However, systematic review done in this regard as early as 2004 and further studies showed that not only were these not causally related to TMD, but "partly protective" for TMD.[37] This systematic review and other literature showed that Angle Class II malocclusion, deep bite, and anterior crossbite were protective for TMD.[6,37] Further, there were no occlusal-functional or tooth-occlusal morphologic factors that had any relationship to TMDs. Another population-based study with a population of more than 4000 patients found that no occlusal factor was significantly associated with frequency of subjective TMD symptoms.[38] Further, these studies revealed that no factors of functional occlusion were associated with TMD signs.[39] There was a slight association with bilateral open bite and TMD signs; however; the prevalence of this malocclusion was extremely rare. It was also not clear if this factor caused TMD signs, or an actual TMD-associated condition caused the malocclusion.[39] Because there is no evidence to date of a causal relationship of developmental, static, or functional malocclusion with TMDs, correction of this type of occlusion with a purpose of preventing or treating TMDs is not literature supported and therefore not warranted.

IATROGENIC OCCLUSAL CHANGES AND TEMPOROMANDIBULAR DISORDER

The current thought process in orofacial pain is that a causal relationship between occlusal interferences and TMDs is at best weak.[40] Some of the older literature does mention claims about iatrogenic factors contributing to TMD.[41] Although it has been proposed in some of the literature that iatrogenically introduced supraocclusion (ie, "high points on a new restoration") can cause dental and muscle pain, further to be relieved by the adjustment of these restorations,[42,43] the most recent literature points in a different direction as well. Well-controlled studies using EMG have shown a reduction in masseteric muscle activity upon the introduction of a "high point."[44–46] In other words, the so-called high point relaxes the muscle as opposed to causing it to spasm. Further, the same studies showed that these "high points" also failed to reduce the pressure-pain threshold. Emerging succinct literature on "high points" show that there is no causal relationship between these and TMDs. However, it must be noted that correction of such high points may be crucial to prevent fracture of tooth structure or restoration and odontogenic pain.

LOSS OF TEETH, LOSS OF POSTERIOR SUPPORT, AND TEMPOROMANDIBULAR DISORDER

In the older traditional literature, loss of teeth/posterior support had been proposed to be linked to TMD.[47–51] These findings were predicated on the assumption that occlusal support, being a crucial factor for efficient chewing, would also play an indirect role in preventing TMD. However, most of the recent literature has debunked this myth. Malocclusion as well as loss of posterior teeth do not contribute to TMD as per this robust literature.[52,53] As a matter of fact, many succinct studies have shown that losing more than 5 posterior teeth was more prevalent in a cohort of patients without TMDs, whereas a much lesser percentage of patients with TMD had actual loss of posterior teeth.[52] Loss of posterior teeth has been shown to be poorly associated and correlated with TMD, and there is poor clinical evidence to relate the two.[52,54,55]

OCCLUSAL SPLINT THERAPY AND TEMPOROMANDIBULAR DISORDER

Occlusal splint therapy (either alone or in combination with other modalities), sometimes called "appliance therapy," traditionally has been used by dentists in an attempt to manage pain and other concomitant symptoms that occur with TMDs.[56–62] Although this technique has been used for several decades with varying apparent success rates, an exact mechanism of if/how they work has not been elucidated. A relatively wide range of theories have been proposed. In general, these appliances, although transiently altering the way teeth come into contact, have been proposed to reduce muscle and joint pain.[63] In the case of myogenous TMD, physical therapy modalities were found to be as effective as occlusal splints.[64] Occlusal splints have also been proposed to affect postural balance.[65] The so-called special splints such as "biofeedback splints" have been claimed to be of some benefit in reducing TMD symptoms.[66] However, systematic reviews have failed to demonstrate any superiority of or distinction from the clinical effectiveness of occlusal splints as compared with exercise therapy in painful TMDs.[67] Another recent network meta-analysis of a large number of randomized controlled trials showed that the evidence confirming the effectiveness of occlusal splints was of very low quality. This study also reported that a combination of hard stabilization splints coupled with counseling therapy was the most beneficial in improving TMD symptomatology in patients.[68] Although dental clinicians seem to prefer specific type of splint material over others, this topic has been controversial. Some studies have shown that hard splints offer faster reduction of symptoms than soft splints.[69] The same literature also showed that both hard and soft splints are equally efficacious. However, more controlled studies with well-thought study design have shown that nonoccluding splints (therefore when the patient closes, the teeth contact in occlusion) were as effective as fully occluding hard or soft splints. The role of occlusion on the splint in symptom reduction is unclear.

TOOTH REPLACEMENT AND TEMPOROMANDIBULAR DISORDER (EDENTULOUS/DENTULOUS)

Although considered the mainstay for "prevention" of TMD in the older dental literature, the current evidence points out that replacement of lost teeth and reestablishment of posterior bite/occlusion are not primarily indicated for preventing TMDs.[70] Further, this type of succinct literature also advocates the prudence of simple, reversible methods in the management of TMDs rather than complex prosthodontic treatment with a view to prevent TMDs, the latter being a fallacy. Most of the consensus in the scientific literature is that generalized prophylactic occlusal adjustments (including occlusal equilibrations) are not justified in the prevention or management of TMDs.[70]

CLINICAL PEARLS

The fundamental principles of dental occlusion derived from the literature and conventional wisdom that have guided dentists over the past several decades are crucial for maintaining and reestablishing a sound stomatognathic system. These principles are incorporated into reconstruction of the bite in order to optimize form and function. These paradigms also are critical in maintaining the integrity of the new occlusion and function that the reconstructive dentist provides their patients. However, the current literature is clear in that following the principles of occlusion has minimal, if anything, to do with prevention of TMD. Reestablishing lost bite or occlusion should not be intended as a measure to prevent development of TMD. Orthodontic or other correction of malocclusion is also not intended to prevent TMD or alleviate TMD symptoms. There is also mounting evidence that noncorrection of occlusal disharmonies fails to initiate TMDs. Further, correction of malocclusion has not shown to delay or prevent TMD or TMD pain. Malocclusion can occur as a sequela of acute or chronic TMD. There is no convincing evidence showing TMD causation or predisposition by a naturally occurring malocclusion in a patient. Correction of a probable coexisting condition with certain skeletal malocclusions (Class II association with obstructive sleep apnea) may be instrumental in reducing or ameliorating signs and symptoms of possible TMD musculoskeletal pain. However, the clinician must take precaution not to associate these TMD pain symptoms to the malocclusion, on the contrary, should look at other factors associated with the primary cause (such as hypoxia). Splint therapy has been shown as a reversible, noninvasive method for management of TMD pain. The exact mechanism of how splints help the patient with TMD is yet to be elucidated.

Contrary to the older literature, loss of posterior teeth/vertical dimension/posterior support does not seem to predispose to or cause TMD. Irreversible occlusal adjustments, such as occlusal equilibration, with a sole purpose of treating sleep-related bruxism is not supported by the current succinct literature. Similarly, there is no reliable evidence that so-called occlusal interferences and eccentricities have any causal relationship with the causation or perpetuation of TMD or TMD symptoms. Therefore, currently there is no justification for removing these interferences with a sole purpose of preventing or ameliorating TMDs. Any observed association of malocclusions such as caused by deep bite or tooth crowding to a coexisting TMD has only the value of an observational study. Therefore, attempts to correct these with a sole purpose of preventing or treating TMDs are not justified by the current sound literature. Further, well-controlled prospective studies with excellent study design and identification of confounders are the need of the time to establish any causal relationship of malocclusion or changes in occlusion to TMD. Until then, irreversible changes iatrogenically inflicted upon naturally occurring dentition with a purpose of treating TMD are not warranted.

DISCLOSURE

D.C. Thomas, S.R. Singer, and S. Markman have no commercial or financial conflicts of interest. No funding was requested or received for this article.

REFERENCES

1. Valesan LF, Da-Cas CD, Réus JC, et al. Prevalence of temporomandibular joint disorders: a systematic review and meta-analysis. Clin Oral Investig 2021; 25(2):441–53.

2. Health UDo, Services H. National Institute of Dental and Craniofacial Research. Oral health in America: a report of the surgeon general. Rockville, MD: US Public Health Service, Department of Health and Human Services; 2000.
3. List T, Jensen RH. Temporomandibular disorders: old ideas and new concepts. Cephalalgia 2017;37(7):692–704.
4. Rosales AS, Rodríguez EAV, González CLL, et al. Association Between -1607 1G/2G Polymorphism of MMP1 and Temporomandibular Joint Anterior Disc Displacement with Reduction. Braz Dent J 2020;31(2):152–6.
5. Young AL. Internal derangements of the temporomandibular joint: a review of the anatomy, diagnosis, and management. J Indian Prosthodont Soc 2015;15(1):2–7.
6. Kalladka M, Young A, Thomas D, et al. The relation of temporomandibular disorders and dental occlusion: a narrative review. Quintessence Int 2022;53(5):450–9.
7. Kang MG, Park YJ, Huh KH, et al. Clinical characteristics of temporomandibular disorders presenting posterior open bite - A report of 12 cases. J Dent Sci 2021; 16(3):861–7.
8. Kato C, Ono T. Anterior open bite due to temporomandibular joint osteoarthrosis with muscle dysfunction treated with temporary anchorage devices. Am J Orthod Dentofacial Orthop 2018;154(6):848–59.
9. Caldas W, Conti AC, Janson G, et al. Occlusal changes secondary to temporomandibular joint conditions: a critical review and implications for clinical practice. J Appl Oral Sci 2016;24(4):411–9.
10. Hirsch C, John MT, Drangsholt MT, et al. Relationship between overbite/overjet and clicking or crepitus of the temporomandibular joint. J Orofac Pain. Summer 2005;19(3):218–25.
11. Kim Y-K. Temporomandibular Joint Disorder and Occlusal Changes. J Korean Dental Sci 2018;11(1):21–31.
12. Okeson JP. Management of temporomandibular disorders and occlusion. 6th edition. Louis, MO: Mosby Elsevier; 2007.
13. Thomas DC, Kohli D, Chen N, et al. Orofacial manifestations of rheumatoid arthritis and systemic lupus erythematosus: a narrative review. Quintessence Int 2021;52(5):454–66.
14. Manfredini D, Castroflorio T, Perinetti G, et al. Dental occlusion, body posture and temporomandibular disorders: where we are now and where we are heading for. J Oral Rehabil 2012;39(6):463–71.
15. Luther F. TMD and occlusion part II. Damned if we don't? Functional occlusal problems: TMD epidemiology in a wider context. Br Dent J 2007;202(1):E3 [discussion: 38-9].
16. Pahkala R, Qvarnström M. Can temporomandibular dysfunction signs be predicted by early morphological or functional variables? Eur J Orthod 2004;26(4): 367–73.
17. Mohlin B, Axelsson S, Paulin G, et al. TMD in relation to malocclusion and orthodontic treatment. Angle Orthod 2007;77(3):542–8.
18. Wang MQ, Cao HT, Liu FR, et al. Association of tightly locked occlusion with temporomandibular disorders. J Oral Rehabil 2007;34(3):169–73.
19. Kahn J, Tallents RH, Katzberg RW, et al. Prevalence of dental occlusal variables and intraarticular temporomandibular disorders: molar relationship, lateral guidance, and nonworking side contacts. J Prosthet Dent 1999;82(4):410–5.
20. Silva PF, Motta LJ, Silva SM, et al. Computerized analysis of the distribution of occlusal contacts in individuals with Parkinson's disease and temporomandibular disorder. Cranio 2016;34(6):358–62.

21. Lauriti L, Motta LJ, de Godoy CH, et al. Influence of temporomandibular disorder on temporal and masseter muscles and occlusal contacts in adolescents: an electromyographic study. BMC Musculoskelet Disord 2014;15:123.
22. John MT, Hirsch C, Drangsholt MT, et al. Overbite and overjet are not related to self-report of temporomandibular disorder symptoms. J Dent Res 2002;81(3):164–9.
23. Kandasamy S, Greene CS, Rinchuse DJ, et al. TMD and orthodontics : a clinical guide for the orthodontist. Switzerland: Springer International Publishing; 2015. https://doi.org/10.1007/978-3-319-19782-1. Available at: https://search.ebscohost.com/login.aspx?direct=true&scope=site&db=nlebk&db=nlabk&AN=1055008 http://www.myilibrary.com?id=825156 https://public.ebookcentral.proquest.com/choice/publicfullrecord.aspx?p=3568681 http://books.scholarsportal.info/viewdoc.html?id=/ebooks/ebooks3/springer/2017-08-17/2/9783319197821 https://link.springer.com/book/10.1007/978-3-319-19781-4 https://link.springer.com/book/10.1007/978-3-319-19782-1 http://www.vlebooks.com/vleweb/product/openreader?id=none&isbn=9783319197821 https://discover.gcu.ac.uk/discovery/openurl?institution=44GLCU_INST&vid=44GLCU_INST:44GLCU_VU2&?u.ignore_date_coverage=true&rft.mms_id=991002484139303836.
24. Pullinger AG, Seligman DA. The degree to which attrition characterizes differentiated patient groups of temporomandibular disorders. J Orofac Pain 1993;7(2):196–208. Spring.
25. Sonnesen L, Bakke M, Solow B. Malocclusion traits and symptoms and signs of temporomandibular disorders in children with severe malocclusion. Eur J Orthod 1998;20(5):543–59.
26. Kecik D, Kocadereli I, Saatci I. Evaluation of the treatment changes of functional posterior crossbite in the mixed dentition. Am J Orthod Dentofacial Orthop 2007;131(2):202–15.
27. Vanderas AP, Papagiannoulis L. Multifactorial analysis of the aetiology of craniomandibular dysfunction in children. Int J Paediatr Dent 2002;12(5):336–46.
28. Andrade Ada S, Gameiro GH, Derossi M, et al. Posterior crossbite and functional changes. A systematic review. Angle Orthod 2009;79(2):380–6.
29. Khayat N, Winocur E, Emodi Perelman A, et al. The prevalence of posterior crossbite, deep bite, and sleep or awake bruxism in temporomandibular disorder (TMD) patients compared to a non-TMD population: a retrospective study. Cranio 2021;39(5):398–404.
30. Khayat N, Winocur E, Kedem R, et al. The prevalence of temporomandibular disorders and dental attrition levels in patients with posterior crossbite and/or deep bite: a preliminary prospective study. Pain Res Manag 2021;2021:8827895.
31. The Glossary of Prosthodontic Terms: Ninth Edition. J Prosthet Dent 2017;117(5s):e1–105.
32. Cao Y, Xie QF, Li K, et al. Experimental occlusal interference induces long-term masticatory muscle hyperalgesia in rats. Pain 2009;144(3):287–93.
33. Clark GT, Tsukiyama Y, Baba K, et al. Sixty-eight years of experimental occlusal interference studies: what have we learned? J Prosthet Dent 1999;82(6):704–13.
34. Landi N, Manfredini D, Tognini F, et al. Quantification of the relative risk of multiple occlusal variables for muscle disorders of the stomatognathic system. J Prosthet Dent 2004;92(2):190–5.
35. Türp JC, Greene CS, Strub JR. Dental occlusion: a critical reflection on past, present and future concepts. J Oral Rehabil 2008;35(6):446–53.
36. Henrikson T, Ekberg EC, Nilner M. Symptoms and signs of temporomandibular disorders in girls with normal occlusion and Class II malocclusion. Acta Odontol Scand 1997;55(4):229–35.

37. Gesch D, Bernhardt O, Kirbschus A. Association of malocclusion and functional occlusion with temporomandibular disorders (TMD) in adults: a systematic review of population-based studies. Quintessence Int 2004;35(3):211–21.
38. Gesch D, Bernhardt O, Mack F, et al. Association of malocclusion and functional occlusion with subjective symptoms of TMD in adults: results of the Study of Health in Pomerania (SHIP). Angle Orthod 2005;75(2):183–90.
39. Gesch D, Bernhardt O, Kocher T, et al. Association of malocclusion and functional occlusion with signs of temporomandibular disorders in adults: results of the population-based study of health in Pomerania. Angle Orthod 2004;74(4): 512–20.
40. Alamir AH, Hakami YA, Alabsi FS, et al. Potential myogenous temporomandibular disorders following iatrogenic occlusal disturbance: a pilot study. J Contemp Dent Pract 2019;20(10):1138–40.
41. Hagag G, Yoshida K, Miura H. Occlusion, prosthodontic treatment, and temporomandibular disorders: a review. J Med Dent Sci 2000;47(1):61–6.
42. Carlsson GE. Dental occlusion: modern concepts and their application in implant prosthodontics. Odontology 2009;97(1):8–17.
43. Johansson A, Johansson AK, Omar R, et al. Rehabilitation of the worn dentition. J Oral Rehabil 2008;35(7):548–66.
44. Minervini G, Romano A, Petruzzi M, et al. Oral-facial-digital syndrome (OFD): 31-year follow-up management and monitoring. J Biol Regul Homeost Agents 2018; 32(2 Suppl. 1):127–30.
45. Minervini G, Russo D, Herford AS, et al. Teledentistry in the Management of Patients with Dental and Temporomandibular Disorders. Biomed Res Int 2022;2022: 7091153.
46. Minervini G, Fiorillo L, Russo D, et al. Prosthodontic treatment in patients with temporomandibular disorders and orofacial pain and/or bruxism: a review of the literature. Prosthesis 2022;4(2):253–62.
47. Ueno M, Yanagisawa T, Shinada K, et al. Category of functional tooth units in relation to the number of teeth and masticatory ability in Japanese adults. Clin Oral Investig 2010;14(1):113–9.
48. Nguyen MS, Jagomägi T, Nguyen T, et al. Occlusal Support and Temporomandibular Disorders Among Elderly Vietnamese. Int J Prosthodont 2017;30(5):465–70.
49. Tallents RH, Macher DJ, Kyrkanides S, et al. Prevalence of missing posterior teeth and intraarticular temporomandibular disorders. J Prosthet Dent 2002;87(1): 45–50.
50. Wang MQ, Xue F, He JJ, et al. Missing posterior teeth and risk of temporomandibular disorders. J Dent Res 2009;88(10):942–5.
51. Ciancaglini R, Gherlone EF, Radaelli G. Association between loss of occlusal support and symptoms of functional disturbances of the masticatory system. J Oral Rehabil 1999;26(3):248–53.
52. de Sousa ST, de Mello VV, Magalhães BG, et al. The role of occlusal factors on the occurrence of temporomandibular disorders. Cranio 2015;33(3):211–6.
53. Nguyen MS, Saag M, Jagomägi T, et al. The impact of occlusal support on temporomandibular disorders: a literature review. Proc Singapore Healthc 2021. https://doi.org/10.1177/20101058211023779.
54. Manfredini D, Perinetti G, Guarda-Nardini L. Dental malocclusion is not related to temporomandibular joint clicking: a logistic regression analysis in a patient population. Angle Orthod 2014;84(2):310–5.
55. Manfredini D, Perinetti G, Stellini E, et al. Prevalence of static and dynamic dental malocclusion features in subgroups of temporomandibular disorder patients:

Implications for the epidemiology of the TMD-occlusion association. Quintessence Int 2015;46(4):341–9.

56. Ekberg EC, Vallon D, Nilner M. Occlusal appliance therapy in patients with temporomandibular disorders. A double-blind controlled study in a short-term perspective. Acta Odontol Scand 1998;56(2):122–8.

57. Ekberg E, Vallon D, Nilner M. The efficacy of appliance therapy in patients with temporomandibular disorders of mainly myogenous origin. A randomized, controlled, short-term trial. J Orofac Pain 2003;17(2):133–9. Spring.

58. Ekberg E, Nilner M. Treatment outcome of appliance therapy in temporomandibular disorder patients with myofascial pain after 6 and 12 months. Acta Odontol Scand 2004;62(6):343–9.

59. Greene CS, Laskin DM. Splint therapy for the myofascial pain–dysfunction (MPD) syndrome: a comparative study. J Am Dent Assoc 1972;84(3):624–8.

60. Fricton J. Current evidence providing clarity in management of temporomandibular disorders: summary of a systematic review of randomized clinical trials for intra-oral appliances and occlusal therapies. J Evid Based Dent Pract 2006;6(1):48–52.

61. Wassell RW, Adams N, Kelly PJ. The treatment of temporomandibular disorders with stabilizing splints in general dental practice: one-year follow-up. J Am Dent Assoc 2006;137(8):1089–98 [quiz: 1168-9].

62. Zhang C, Wu JY, Deng DL, et al. Efficacy of splint therapy for the management of temporomandibular disorders: a meta-analysis. Oncotarget 2016;7(51):84043–53.

63. Kümbüloğlu O, Saracoglu A, Bingöl P, et al. Clinical study on the comparison of masticatory efficiency and jaw movement before and after temporomandibular disorder treatment. Cranio 2013;31(3):190–201.

64. van Grootel RJ, Buchner R, Wismeijer D, et al. Towards an optimal therapy strategy for myogenous TMD, physiotherapy compared with occlusal splint therapy in an RCT with therapy-and-patient-specific treatment durations. BMC Musculoskelet Disord 2017;18(1):76.

65. Oliveira SSI, Pannuti CM, Paranhos KS, et al. Effect of occlusal splint and therapeutic exercises on postural balance of patients with signs and symptoms of temporomandibular disorder. Clin Exp Dent Res 2019;5(2):109–15.

66. Bergmann A, Edelhoff D, Schubert O, et al. Effect of treatment with a full-occlusion biofeedback splint on sleep bruxism and TMD pain: a randomized controlled clinical trial. Clin Oral Investig 2020;24(11):4005–18.

67. Zhang L, Xu L, Wu D, et al. Effectiveness of exercise therapy versus occlusal splint therapy for the treatment of painful temporomandibular disorders: a systematic review and meta-analysis. Ann Palliat Med 2021;10(6):6122–32.

68. Al-Moraissi EA, Farea R, Qasem KA, et al. Effectiveness of occlusal splint therapy in the management of temporomandibular disorders: network meta-analysis of randomized controlled trials. Int J Oral Maxillofac Surg 2020;49(8):1042–56.

69. Poorna TA, John B, Joshna EK, et al. Comparison of the effectiveness of soft and hard splints in the symptomatic management of temporomandibular joint disorders: a randomized control study. Int J Rheum Dis 2022;25(9):1053–9.

70. De Boever JA, Carlsson GE, Klineberg IJ. Need for occlusal therapy and prosthodontic treatment in the management of temporomandibular disorders. Part II: Tooth loss and prosthodontic treatment. J Oral Rehabil 2000;27(8):647–59.

Temporomandibular Disorders
Implications in Restorative Dentistry and Orthodontics

Davis C. Thomas, BDS, DDS, MSD, MSc Med, MSc[a,b,]*, David Briss, DMD[c],
Paul Emile Rossouw, MChD, PhD[d], Shankar Iyer, DDS, MDS[e,f,g]

KEYWORDS

- Temporomandibular disorders ● Full-mouth rehabilitations ● Orthodontic treatment
- Prosthodontic treatment ● Occlusion ● Restorative dentistry ● Malocclusion

KEY POINTS

- The health of the temporomandibular joint (TMJ) and associated structures are paramount for optimal results from orthodontic and prosthodontic/restorative treatment.
- The clinician contemplating orthodontic and restorative treatment should be prudent in checking for any preexisting temporomandibular disorder (TMD) issues before initiation of treatment. It is essential for the clinician to have a clear understanding of screening for health of the TMJ and associated structures. This would facilitate prompt referral to the appropriate specialist before the start of orthodontic/restorative treatment.
- There is no succinct evidence of orthodontic or prosthodontic treatment (or lack thereof) causing TMD.
- There is an immense need for well-controlled, double-blinded prospective studies exploring any possible association between orthodontic/prosthodontic treatment and TMD.

---

[a] Department of Diagnostic Sciences, Rutgers School of Dental Medicine, 110 Bergen Street, Newark, NJ 07103, USA; [b] Eastman Institute of Oral Health, Rochester, NY, USA; [c] Department of Orthodontics, Rutgers School of Dental Medicine, 110 Bergen Street, Newark, NJ 07103, USA; [d] Department of Orthodontics and Dentofacial Orthopedics, Eastman Institute for Oral Health, University of Rochester, 625 Elmwood Avenue, Box 683, Rochester, NY 14620, USA; [e] Private Practice limited to Prosthodontics, Elizabeth, NJ, USA; [f] Department of Prosthodontics, Rutgers University, 110 Bergen Street, Newark, NJ 07103, USA; [g] Department of Periodontics, Rutgers University, 110 Bergen Street, Newark, NJ 07103, USA
* Corresponding author. Department of Diagnostic Sciences, Rutgers School of Dental Medicine, 110 Bergen Street, Newark, NJ 07103.
E-mail address: davisct1@gmail.com

Dent Clin N Am 67 (2023) 309–321
https://doi.org/10.1016/j.cden.2022.10.003
0011-8532/23/© 2023 Elsevier Inc. All rights reserved.

INTRODUCTION

Dentists traditionally have always looked for guidance as to the principles of orthodontic treatment and prosthodontic reconstruction, specifically with a view to avoid "causing" temporomandibular disorders (TMDs). Various philosophies have been proposed, many of them apparently based on hypotheses and personal observations. Well-controlled, prospective double-blinded studies regarding the causality (or lack thereof) of TMDs secondary to changes in the bite/occlusion as a result of reconstructive dental management are lacking. For example, in the early pioneer orthodontic literature, dental occlusion was classified into Class I, II, and III based on certain factors that angle observed in the population at which he was looking. However, during the subsequent decades, this observation that he made probably was misinterpreted and TMDs were apparently erroneously attributed to malocclusion. Similarly, in prosthodontics and reconstructive dentistry, certain changes in the patient's occlusion, by virtue of dental treatment, was thought of as causally related to TMDs. The relation between occlusion and TMDs is explored in a separate chapter in this special edition. In this article, the authors enumerate the literature on the current thought process in orthodontic management and prosthodontics as related to TMDs.

Temporomandibular Disorder and Orthodontics

According to the overwhelming orthodontic and TMD literature, occlusal disharmonies and most maxillomandibular relationships have no causality to the development of TMD symptoms.[1-5] The coincidence between the age groups, namely adolescents, of orthodontic treatment and TMD may become challenging for the orthodontist, although it may be difficult to figure out which of the two entities came first. It is suggested that it would be prudent to postpone orthodontic treatment and address the TMD issue. Then, orthodontic treatment can be resumed.[6] Various protocols based on hypotheses including centric relation (CR) position, "deprogramming," neuromuscular dentistry, jaw tracking, electromyographic recording, and preventive occlusal equilibrations have been proposed by various professionals and organizations in an attempt to optimize dental/orthodontic treatment. However, most of the published scientific literature contradicts the use of these philosophies and criticizes the invasive and irreversible nature of many of these procedures. Further, they are considered to be highly biased and arbitrary.[6-11]

Similar to this myth is the one that said that the so-called Class II malocclusion is related to TMD.[12-14] There was no such relationship found between Class II malocclusion and TMD in multiple studies/literature published.[2,15-17] Further, there was no association found between horizontal/vertical dental relationship of the anterior teeth and temporomandibular joint (TMJ) disc derangements.[18-20] The concept of occlusion as an etiology for overloading of the masticatory system has been popular among various dental groups, including some orthodontists.[21] It must be pointed out, however, that considering the continuous dynamic change that occurs during several months of orthodontic treatment, there is hardly any evidence for development of TMDs. In the context of sleep-related bruxism (SRB), the status of the current literature is relatively clear that orthodontic treatment affecting in SRB in any way, is yet to be elucidated. Currently, the literature seems to indicate that orthodontic treatment has no significant effect on SRB.[22,23] As alluded to earlier, orthodontic treatment aimed at "correcting a patient's occlusion" into a "proper" CR position, is currently not believed to be of any meaningful significance.[24,25] Similarly, the philosophy of "failure to achieve functional occlusion/CR," forming an etiology for TMD is also thought to be of no scientific evidence.[26–29] Recent multiple studies and publications have shown that neither does dental occlusion have any causal role in the etiopathophysiology of TMD, nor the correction of the same by orthodontics can meaningfully treat or prevent TMD.[30–32]

It must be noted that a few studies, some of them recent, have stated a "higher prevalence" of TMD with orthodontically treated patients, however, explicitly stating that a cause-effect relationship between orthodontic treatment and TMD could not be established.[33] A few reported orthodontic parameters that were apparently linked with TMD included, but not limited to, a higher Frankfort-mandibular plane angle, increased anterior facial height, increased gonial angle, and Class III malocclusion[34,35] Other general parameters proposed to have an association with TMD included untreated crossbite, dental crowding, increased overjet, condylar asymmetry, long facial height, and a skeletal pattern that is hyperdivergent.[3,36,37] Some investigators have proposed that establishment of a flat occlusal plane is a significant end-result parameter when considering orthodontic treatment, in an attempt to preserve the health and structure of TMJ and associated structures.[38]

The proposal/hypothesis that orthodontic treatment could prevent or alleviate TMD is largely based on the philosophy that malposition of the jaws and teeth are causally related to TMD. Consequently, some of the orthodontic approaches have proposed that when the concepts of "functional occlusion" are "violated," it becomes a trigger for development of TMD.[39,40] The older concept/hypothesis of TMD being caused by specific orthodontic modalities and the retraction of maxillary incisor teeth ("causing condylar distalization and anterior disc displacement") has been negated substantially by the more recent orthodontic/TMD literature.[3,22,40–43] In addition, the previous concepts of TMD causation by the use of "chin cup therapy" for Class III malocclusion correction to be causing TMD has also been disproven in imaging-based studies.[44] It must be noted that recent literature has overwhelmingly debunked the older concepts of the so-called principles of gnathology that proposed occlusion and malocclusion as linked to TMD.[3,22,40–43] Further, robust evidence in the literature refutes any association of corrective orthodontic treatment to an increase/decrease in the risk of an individual developing TMD due to any orthodontic treatment.[40,45]

Another interesting proposed concept is that stability of the condyles and the occlusion "reduces the risk of TMD." The clinician should assess and manage this aspect before orthodontic intervention.[46] Meanwhile, other published papers have described the concept of "adaptation" to occlusal changes in orthodontic treatment without any measurable TMD.[47] Observational studies and smaller cohort studies have reported milder transient TMD symptoms occurring with orthodontic treatment.[39] There have been other hypotheses and proposals linking what is termed as transverse malocclusions to "uneven loading" of the TMJ.[39] TMD symptoms have also been reported to be associated with orthognathic surgeries.[48] Transient masticatory muscle pain was also reported more often in females undergoing orthodontic treatments compared with males.[1] Most of these studies and published papers conclude universally by saying that further, well-controlled, prospective studies are necessary for elucidating the link between any of these factors with TMD.

Association of Temporomandibular Disorder and Prosthodontics

One of the first references in the published literature is from Costen, where he hypothesized that when that a loss of vertical dimension caused by tooth loss and a subsequent collapsed facial profile, it leads to tinnitus.[49] The profession was awakened by this newfound etiology for ear, nose, and throat abnormalities. This was further explored by Hirschfeld, who attributed "over 80 changes" that can occur from the loss of the first molar, TMJ changes being one of them.[50] We explore the dogmas that have been prevalent in prosthetic dentistry and will attempt to clarify some of these controversies based on scientific evidence. The following are some of the concepts that will be discussed to question the practices that have steered practitioners into various philosophies that may have locked them into a particular apparently inflexible approach.

1. Do occlusal interferences and "high points" cause muscle hyperactivity and precipitate TMD?
2. Can altering a patient's vertical dimension precipitate TMD symptoms?
3. Can gnathological principles protect a patient from developing TMD (Is it necessary to follow principles of "gnathology" to obtain correct occlusal schemes)?
4. Should every prosthodontic rehabilitation end up in a Class I relationship?
5. Are occlusal reconstructions a way to mitigate the symptoms of TMD?

Do occlusal interferences and "high points" cause muscle hyperactivity and precipitate temporomandibular disorder?

A flawed understanding of etiology has kept in the subsequent treatment rendered. In this regard, it must be borne in mind that occlusal interferences have not been considered as one of the etiologic factors for TMD for a long time in literature. Although some investigators have attempted to elicit the role of occlusion in TMD via some electromyogram (EMG) studies,[51] numerous contributors have negated that viewpoint. Weinberg (1979) in a three-part series article attributed the etiology of TMD symptoms to multiple causes, including neurologic, vascular, the TMJ itself, muscular, and hysterical conversion ("psychogenic?"). Clearly, "bad occlusion" or occlusal interferences were not accounted for as a causative factor for TMD.[52–54]

Deliberate introduction of interferences in a group of patients failed to show an obligatory relationship with TMD. These clinical results have been backed by EMG findings as well.[55–57]

Contrary reports by investigators have also been documented in the literature.[58] However, with mounting evidence in the literature failing to find that occlusal disharmony causes any long-term deleterious effects on TMJ, it can be concluded that indiscriminate adjustment of occlusion can probably do greater irreversible harm than good in the long run, and practitioners should be cautious to implement any irreversible changes without a sound scientific backing.[32,59–62] In fact, occlusal changes secondary to changes in the joint is also a possibility and may manifest, either as a momentary event or as a prolonged condition.[31,32,63–66]

Can altering a patient's vertical dimension precipitate temporomandibular disorder symptoms?

A relatively recent literature review concluded that there is very little or weak correlation between altering the occlusal vertical dimension (OVD) and initiation of TMD symptoms.[67] Further, this article also alludes to the fact that there is a lack of well-controlled studies in this regard.[67] Multiple studies that looked at the effect of increasing OVD failed to show any correlation or causality with TMD symptoms.[68–72] Similarly, other studies including prospective have also shown that reduction in the vertical dimension, whether brought about by attrition, erosion, or loss of teeth, is not correlated or causally related to long-lasting TMD signs and symptoms.[67,73] Tooth wear/loss or changes in the existing prostheses over time are the clinical conditions that may demand increasing the patient's existing OVD.[74] It is well documented in the scientific literature that making changes in OVD is a safe and predictable procedure, without detrimental consequences, as long as physiologic tolerance is not challenged.[75,76] A relatively recent review of the literature concluded that there is very little or weak correlation between altering vertical dimension and TMD symptoms.[67] These investigators opine that the basis of the theory that increasing OVD causing TMD is anecdotal or just solitary case reports and not evidence-based. In fact, they suggest that the moderate changes in stomatognathic system tend toward adaptation.[67] It is noteworthy that unfavorable consequences that have been documented in a few studies due to increase in OVD are transient and self-limiting.[77,78] Therefore, it has been suggested that irreversible alteration in the occlusion should be preceded by the use of a reversible occlusal appliance to give the patient time to adapt to the change in vertical dimension. Most of the data from studies support the fact that the stomatognathic system has the ability to adapt quickly to moderate changes in OVD of less than 5 mm, with orthopedic stability being maintained.[67] It must be emphasized that in the pretext of preventing TMD, occlusal therapy and full-mouth rehabilitation should not be promoted for conditions such as bruxism, erosion, and parafunctional habits.[79]

Can gnathological principles protect a patient from developing temporomandibular disorder (is it necessary to follow principles of "gnathology" to obtain correct occlusal schemes)?

Occlusion in prosthodontics became mechanically-based since the birth of gnathology in the early 1920s.[80–83] The articulators evolved and got more sophisticated and there were developers trying to mimic the mandibular movements.[84–87] The carvings of the occlusion were mechanically and geometrically determined, defined by angles and arcs created by pantographs and jaw tracking devices.[88] Later, however, it was concluded that these rigid gnathological standards were not based on scientific grounds and the concept of "ideal occlusion" was no more than a result of individual observations and should not be considered as a synonym for physiologic occlusion.[89–93]

In fact, Mohl negated that attempts to develop "ideal occlusion" by mechanics following rigid occlusal schemes in otherwise well-functioning patients were not always tolerated by the patient, despite the adaptive potential of TMJ.[94] The concept of "point centric" with no freedom in lateral or anterior to the point was strongly negated, and concept of functionally optimal occlusion was appreciated.[36,42,43] Celenza's treatise on CR as a treatment position, and not a position of constancy was met with much skepticism.[95] By the 1990s, the use of sophisticated fully adjustable articulators was slowly diminishing in specialty practice, and the gnathological concepts gave way to simpler practical facial analyzers and average settings on semi-adjustable articulators.[96]

Despite ample evidence that occlusion plays a limited role in influencing TMD, neuromuscular dentistry and other bio-functional concepts continue to be fostered by certain groups of dentists. There are no randomized control trials to verify if any of these have worked consistently and remains as anecdotal evidence.[79]

Should every prosthodontic rehabilitation end up in a Class I relationship?

Seligman and Pullinger evaluated conditions such as deep bite, overjet, crossbite, and open bites and found no correlation between any of the occlusal interrelationships and TMD.[97]

In restorative dentistry, a deliberate attempt to create anterior guidance has been the mainstay with natural teeth and implants. It has been traditionally proposed that to achieve a mutually protected occlusal scheme, cases have to be restored in a Class I relationship. The fallacy of a normal Class I relationship as being ideal can be questioned by the racial distribution of the occlusal schemes around the world. If Class I occlusion is the ideal tooth relationship, we would have seen an explosion of TMD cases in populations where Class III occlusion is a normal finding. In fact, it has been demonstrated by numerous investigators that the prevalence of malocclusions is the same in populations with TMD and in the general population and there is no association between risk of developing TMD and occlusal characteristics.[3,5,26,31,32,98–106]

Are occlusal reconstructions a way to mitigate the symptoms of temporomandibular disorder?

There are several conditions such as bruxism, erosion, and parafunctional habits that may cause tooth wear and other types of tooth loss. Full-mouth rehabilitation and occlusal therapy should not be promoted as a means of preventing TMD, as there is no evidence of the benefits or necessity for this type of seemingly aggressive management.

Centric Relation

There is no real evidence of condylar positioning in the glenoid fossa having any causality for initiation of TMD.[40,107–109] Further, none of the traditionally described ways of registering a so-called "stable centric relation position" has been proven to be foolproof and evidence-based. As a matter of fact, imaging-based studies have shown that all of the procedures looked at, are in effect "blind procedures" and unable to independently repeat and verify.[110,111] It also must be noted that numerous publications have successfully questioned the accuracy and repeatability of such recording instruments as facebows, tracings, articulators, and condylar position indicators, basically due to the multitude of possible errors[112,113] Concepts of TMD, as related to orthodontics, has been drastically changed over the last few decades, basically due to succinct science and evidence-based approaches of looking at the validity of the philosophies and the approaches that have evolved during this period. This drastic change has been catalyzed by advances in the fields of pain management, pain pathophysiology and neurophysiology, genetics, principles of physiatry, behavioral and psychological sciences, and orthopedics. The older rigid mechanical models of TMJ and the dependent TMD literature are being overwhelmingly debunked. A new era of the biopsychosocial model of orofacial pain in general, and TMD in particular, has risen. The relatively crude anecdotal literature of orthodontic treatment as a cause of TMD is largely disappearing. It is our opinion based on evidence, science, and literature that sound management principles of restorative dentistry and orthodontics have no etiology in causing TMDs and will continue to drive restorative dentistry and orthodontics into a new century.

Clinical Pearls

With all the advances in the fields of orthodontics and prosthodontics/restorative dentistry, one of the areas our field of dentistry is lacking, is the question of any association of these treatment modalities to TMD. The astute clinician must educate himself/herself to screen for TMD issues before initiating orthodontic correction or prosthodontic/restorative intervention. Prompt referral to an orofacial pain specialist or a clinician well-versed in the management of TMDs may be a prudent step if the screening is positive for TMD signs and symptoms. There is no evidence found in the literature hitherto published, establishing any level of causal relationship between orthodontic–prosthodontic–restorative treatment to TMD. Conversely, there is little/no evidence linking occlusion, interferences, loss of vertical dimension, malocclusions, or occlusal prematurities to TMDs. The use of so-called ancillary testing devices such as jaw tracking, kinesiography, total occlusal equilibration, and many other anecdotal principles seem to have little or no evidence in the literature published to date. The traditional principles of prosthodontic reconstruction, orthodontic treatment, and restorative dentistry, including sound occlusal principles, should be followed in an attempt to stabilize the patient's occlusion and optimize esthetics and function.

DISCLOSURE

D.C. Thomas, D. Briss, P.E. Rossouw, and S. Iyer have no commercial or financial conflicts of interest. No funding was received for this article.

REFERENCES

1. Mušanović A, Ajanović M, Redžepagić Vražalica L, et al. Prevalence of TMD among Children Provided with Fixed Orthodontic Treatment. Acta Stomatol Croat 2021;55(2):159–67.
2. McNamara JA Jr, Seligman DA, Okeson JP. Occlusion, Orthodontic treatment, and temporomandibular disorders: a review. J Orofac Pain 1995;9(1):73–90.
3. Michelotti A, Iodice G. The role of orthodontics in temporomandibular disorders. J Oral Rehabil 2010;37(6):411–29.
4. Luther F, Layton S, McDonald F. Orthodontics for treating temporomandibular joint (TMJ) disorders. Cochrane Database Syst Rev 2010;(7):Cd006541. https://doi.org/10.1002/14651858.CD006541.pub2.
5. Egermark I, Magnusson T, Carlsson GE. A 20-year follow-up of signs and symptoms of temporomandibular disorders and malocclusions in subjects with and without orthodontic treatment in childhood. Angle Orthod 2003;73(2):109–15.
6. Kandasamy S, Greene CS, Rinchuse DJ, et al. TMD and Orthodontics A clinical guide for the orthodontist. 1st ed. Springer International Publishing; 2015.
7. Klasser GD, Okeson JP. The clinical usefulness of surface electromyography in the diagnosis and treatment of temporomandibular disorders. J Am Dent Assoc 2006;137(6):763–71.
8. Al-Saleh MA, Armijo-Olivo S, Flores-Mir C, et al. Electromyography in diagnosing temporomandibular disorders. J Am Dent Assoc 2012;143(4):351–62.
9. Manfredini D, Cocilovo F, Favero L, et al. Surface electromyography of jaw muscles and kinesiographic recordings: diagnostic accuracy for myofascial pain. J Oral Rehabil 2011;38(11):791–9.
10. Gonzalez YM, Greene CS, Mohl ND. Technological devices in the diagnosis of temporomandibular disorders. Oral Maxillofacial Surg Clin N Am 2008;20(2): 211–20, vi.
11. Sharma S, Crow HC, McCall WD Jr, et al. Systematic review of reliability and diagnostic validity of joint vibration analysis for diagnosis of temporomandibular disorders. J Orofac Pain 2013;27(1):51–60.
12. Seligman DA, Pullinger AG. Association of occlusal variables among refined TM patient diagnostic groups. J Craniomandib Disord 1989;3(4):227–36.
13. Solberg WK, Bibb CA, Nordström BB, et al. Malocclusion associated with temporomandibular joint changes in young adults at autopsy. Am J Orthod 1986;89(4):326–30.
14. Celić R, Jerolimov V. Association of horizontal and vertical overlap with prevalence of temporomandibular disorders. J Oral Rehabil 2002;29(6):588–93.

15. Dworkin SF, Huggins KH, LeResche L, et al. Epidemiology of signs and symptoms in temporomandibular disorders: clinical signs in cases and controls. J Am Dent Assoc 1990;120(3):273–81.

16. De Boever JA, Adriaens PA. Occlusal relationship in patients with pain-dysfunction symptoms in the temporomandibular joints. J Oral Rehabil 1983; 10(1):1–7.

17. Stringert HG, Worms FW. Variations in skeletal and dental patterns in patients with structural and functional alterations of the temporomandibular joint: a preliminary report. Am J Orthod 1986;89(4):285–97.

18. Ronquillo HI, Guay J, Tallents RH, et al. Comparison of internal derangements with condyle-fossa relationships, horizontal and vertical overlap, and Angle Class. J Craniomandib Disord 1988;2(3):137–40.

19. Pullinger AG, Seligman DA. Overbite and overjet characteristics of refined diagnostic groups of temporomandibular disorder patients. Am J Orthod Dentofacial Orthop 1991;100(5):401–15.

20. John MT, Hirsch C, Drangsholt MT, et al. Overbite and overjet are not related to self-report of temporomandibular disorder symptoms. J Dent Res 2002;81(3): 164–9.

21. Roth RH, Rolfs DA. Functional occlusion for the orthodontist. Part II. J Clin Orthod 1981;15(2):100–23.

22. Hirsch C. No increased risk of temporomandibular disorders and bruxism in children and adolescents during orthodontic therapy. J Orofac Orthop 2009; 70(1):39–50.

23. Fujita Y, Motegi E, Nomura M, et al. Oral habits of temporomandibular disorder patients with malocclusion. Bull Tokyo Dent Coll 2003;44(4):201–7.

24. Derwich M, Pawlowska E. Do the Mandibular Condyles Change Their Positions within Glenoid Fossae after Occlusal Splint Therapy Combined with Physiotherapy in Patients Diagnosed with Temporomandibular Joint Disorders? A Prospective Case Control Study. J Pers Med 2022;(2):12. https://doi.org/10.3390/jpm12020254.

25. Pameijer JH, Brion M, Glickman I, et al. Intraoral occlusal telemetry. V. Effect of occlusal adjustment upon tooth contacts during chewing and swallowing. J Prosthet Dent 1970;24(5):492–7.

26. Gesch D, Bernhardt O, Kirbschus A. Association of malocclusion and functional occlusion with temporomandibular disorders (TMD) in adults: a systematic review of population-based studies. Quintessence Int 2004;35(3):211–21.

27. Mohl ND. Temporomandibular disorders: the role of occlusion, TMJ imaging, and electronic devices. A diagnostic update. J Am Coll Dent 1991;58(3):4–10.

28. Rinchuse DJ, McMinn JT. Summary of evidence-based systematic reviews of temporomandibular disorders. Am J Orthod Dentofacial Orthop 2006;130(6): 715–20.

29. De Kanter RJ, Truin GJ, Burgersdijk RC, et al. Prevalence in the Dutch adult population and a meta-analysis of signs and symptoms of temporomandibular disorder. J Dent Res 1993;72(11):1509–18.

30. Kapos FP, Exposto FG, Oyarzo JF, et al. Temporomandibular disorders: a review of current concepts in aetiology, diagnosis and management. Oral Surg 2020; 13(4):321–34.

31. Manfredini D. Occlusal Equilibration for the Management of Temporomandibular Disorders. Oral Maxillofacial Surg Clin N Am 2018;30(3):257–64.

32. Manfredini D, Lombardo L, Siciliani G. Temporomandibular disorders and dental occlusion. A systematic review of association studies: end of an era? J Oral Rehabil 2017;44(11):908–23.
33. Liu JQ, Wan YD, Xie T, et al. Associations among Orthodontic History, Psychological Status, and Temporomandibular-Related Quality of Life: A Cross-Sectional Study. Int J Clin Pract 2022;2022:3840882.
34. Yan ZB, Wan YD, Xiao CQ, et al. Craniofacial Morphology of Orthodontic Patients with and without Temporomandibular Disorders: A Cross-Sectional Study. Pain Res Manag 2022;2022:9344028.
35. Dygas S, Szarmach I, Radej I. Assessment of the Morphology and Degenerative Changes in the Temporomandibular Joint Using CBCT according to the Orthodontic Approach: A Scoping Review. Biomed Res Int 2022;2022:6863014.
36. Sfondrini MF, Bolognesi L, Bosco M, et al. Skeletal Divergence and Condylar Asymmetry in Patients with Temporomandibular Disorders (TMD): A Retrospective Study. Biomed Res Int 2021;2021:8042910.
37. Dadgar-Yeganeh A, Hatcher DC, Oberoi S. Association between degenerative temporomandibular joint disorders, vertical facial growth, and airway dimension. J World Fed Orthod 2021;10(1):20–8.
38. Buranastidporn B, Hisano M, Soma K. Effect of biomechanical disturbance of the temporomandibular joint on the prevalence of internal derangement in mandibular asymmetry. Eur J Orthod 2006;28(3):199–205.
39. Michelotti A, Rongo R, D'Antò V, et al. Occlusion, orthodontics, and temporomandibular disorders: Cutting edge of the current evidence. J World Fed Orthod 2020;9(3s):S15–8.
40. Kandasamy S, Greene CS. The evolution of temporomandibular disorders: A shift from experience to evidence. J Oral Pathol Med 2020;49(6):461–9.
41. Gianelly AA. Orthodontics, condylar position, and TMJ status. Am J Orthod Dentofacial Orthop 1989;95(6):521–3.
42. Gianelly AA, Anderson CK, Boffa J. Longitudinal evaluation of condylar position in extraction and nonextraction treatment. Am J Orthod Dentofacial Orthop 1991;100(5):416–20.
43. Kim MR, Graber TM, Viana MA. Orthodontics and temporomandibular disorder: a meta-analysis. Am J Orthod Dentofacial Orthop 2002;121(5):438–46.
44. Gökalp H, Arat M, Erden I. The changes in temporomandibular joint disc position and configuration in early orthognathic treatment: a magnetic resonance imaging evaluation. Eur J Orthod 2000;22(3):217–24.
45. Manfredini D, Stellini E, Gracco A, et al. Orthodontics is temporomandibular disorder-neutral. Angle Orthod 2016;86(4):649–54.
46. Karkazi F, Özdemir F. Temporomandibular Disorders: Fundamental Questions and Answers. Turk J Orthod 2020;33(4):246–52.
47. Goodacre CJ, Roberts WE, Goldstein G, et al. Does the Stomatognathic System Adapt to Changes in Occlusion? Best Evidence Consensus Statement. J Prosthodont 2020. https://doi.org/10.1111/jopr.13310.
48. Abrahamsson C. Masticatory function and temporomandibular disorders in patients with dentofacial deformities. Swed Dent J Suppl 2013;231:9–85.
49. Costen JBI. A syndrome of ear and sinus symptoms dependent upon disturbed function of the temporomandibular joint. Ann Otol Rhinol Laryngol 1934;43(1):1–15.
50. Hirschfeld I. The individual missing tooth: a factor in dental and periodontal disease. J Am Dental Assoc Dental Cosmos 1937;24(1):67–82.

51. Karppinen K, Eklund S, Suoninen E, et al. Adjustment of dental occlusion in treatment of chronic cervicobrachial pain and headache. J Oral Rehabil 1999; 26(9):715–21.
52. Weinberg LA. The etiology, diagnosis, and treatment of TMJ dysfunction-pain syndrome. Part I: Etiology. J Prosthet Dent 1979;42(6):654–64.
53. Weinberg LA. Role of condylar position in TMJ dysfunction-pain syndrome. J Prosthet Dent 1979;41(6):636–43.
54. Weinberg LA. An evaluation of occlusal factors in TMJ dysfunction-pain syndrome. J Prosthet Dent 1979;41(2):198–208.
55. Magnusson T, Enbom L. Signs and symptoms of mandibular dysfunction after introduction of experimental balancing-side interferences. Acta Odontol Scand 1984;42(3):129–35.
56. Michelotti A, Farella M, Gallo LM, et al. Effect of occlusal interference on habitual activity of human masseter. J Dent Res 2005;84(7):644–8.
57. Droukas B, Lindée C, Carlsson GE. Relationship between occlusal factors and signs and symptoms of mandibular dysfunction. A clinical study of 48 dental students. Acta Odontol Scand 1984;42(5):277–83.
58. Kirveskari P, Alanen P, Jämsä T. Association between craniomandibular disorders and occlusal interferences in children. J Prosthet Dent 1992;67(5):692–6.
59. Christensen LV, Rassouli NM. Experimental occlusal interferences. Part I. A review. J Oral Rehabil 1995;22(7):515–20.
60. Greene CS. The etiology of temporomandibular disorders: implications for treatment. J Orofac Pain 2001;15(2):93–105, discussion 106-16.
61. Yatani H, Studts J, Cordova M, et al. Comparison of sleep quality and clinical and psychologic characteristics in patients with temporomandibular disorders. J Orofac Pain 2002;16(3):221–8.
62. Koh H, Robinson PG. Occlusal adjustment for treating and preventing temporomandibular joint disorders. J Oral Rehabil 2004;31(4):287–92.
63. Marinho LH, McLoughlin PM. Lateral open bite resulting from acute temporomandibular joint effusion. Br J Oral Maxillofac Surg 1994;32(2):127–8.
64. Pullinger AG, Seligman DA, Gornbein JA. A multiple logistic regression analysis of the risk and relative odds of temporomandibular disorders as a function of common occlusal features. J Dent Res 1993;72(6):968–79.
65. Obrez A, Stohler CS. Jaw muscle pain and its effect on gothic arch tracings. J Prosthet Dent 1996;75(4):393–8.
66. Kalladka M, Young A, Thomas D, et al. The relation of temporomandibular disorders and dental occlusion: a narrative review. Quintessence Int 2022;53(5): 450–9.
67. Moreno-Hay I, Okeson JP. Does altering the occlusal vertical dimension produce temporomandibular disorders? A literature review. J Oral Rehabil 2015; 42(11):875–82.
68. Carlsson GE, Ingervall B, Kocak G. Effect of increasing vertical dimension on the masticatory system in subjects with natural teeth. J Prosthet Dent 1979; 41(3):284–9.
69. Dahl BL, Krogstad O. The effect of a partial bite raising splint on the occlusal face height. An x-ray cephalometric study in human adults. Acta Odontol Scand 1982;40(1):17–24.
70. Dahl BL, Krogstad O. Long-term observations of an increased occlusal face height obtained by a combined orthodontic/prosthetic approach. J Oral Rehabil 1985;12(2):173–6.

71. Gross MD, Ormianer Z. A preliminary study on the effect of occlusal vertical dimension increase on mandibular postural rest position. Int J Prosthodont 1994;7(3):216–26.

72. Ormianer Z, Gross M. A 2-year follow-up of mandibular posture following an increase in occlusal vertical dimension beyond the clinical rest position with fixed restorations. J Oral Rehabil 1998;25(11):877–83.

73. Pullinger AG, Seligman DA. The degree to which attrition characterizes differentiated patient groups of temporomandibular disorders. J Orofac Pain 1993;7(2): 196–208.

74. Goldstein G, Goodacre C, MacGregor K. Occlusal Vertical Dimension: Best Evidence Consensus Statement. J Prosthodont 2021;30(S1):12–9.

75. Abduo J. Safety of increasing vertical dimension of occlusion: a systematic review. Quintessence Int 2012;43(5):369–80.

76. Calamita M, Coachman C, Sesma N, et al. Occlusal vertical dimension: treatment planning decisions and management considerations. Int J Esthet Dent 2019;14(2):166–81.

77. Riise C, Sheikholeslam A. Influence of experimental interfering occlusal contacts on the activity of the anterior temporal and masseter muscles during mastication. J Oral Rehabil 1984;11(4):325–33.

78. Riise C, Sheikholeslam A. The influence of experimental interfering occlusal contacts on the postural activity of the anterior temporal and masseter muscles in young adults. J Oral Rehabil 1982;9(5):419–25.

79. Türp JC, Greene CS, Strub JR. Dental occlusion: a critical reflection on past, present and future concepts. J Oral Rehabil 2008;35(6):446–53.

80. Ash MM Jr. Philosophy of occlusion: past and present. Dent Clin North Am 1995; 39(2):233–55.

81. Stuart C, Golden I. The History of Gnathology, Stuart CE. Gnathological Instr 1981;13-32:113.

82. Brace CL. Occlusion to the anthropological eye. Biol Occlusal Development 1977;7:179–209.

83. Wilson GH. The anatomy and physics of the temporomandibular joint. J Natl Dental Assoc 1921;8(3):236–41.

84. Weinberg LA. An evaluation of basic articulators and their concepts: Part I. Basic concepts. J Prosthet Dent 1963;13(4):622–44.

85. Weinberg LA. An evaluation of basic articulators and their concepts: Part II. Arbitrary, positional, semi adjustable articulators. J Prosthet Dent 1963;13(4): 645–63.

86. Weinberg LA. An evaluation of basic articulators and their concepts: Part IV. Fully adjustable articulators. J Prosthet Dent 1963;13(6):1038–54.

87. Weinberg LA. An evaluation of basic articulators and their concepts: Part III. Fully adjustable articulators. J Prosthet Dent 1963;13(5):873–88.

88. Beyron H. Occlusion: point of significance in planning restorative procedures. J Prosthet Dent 1973;30:641–52.

89. Walther W. Determinants of a healthy aging dentition: maximum number of bilateral centric stops and optimum vertical dimension of occlusion. Int J Prosthodont 2003;16(Suppl):77–9, discussion 89-90.

90. Woda A. A step toward setting norms: comments on the occlusal interface. Int J Prosthodont 2005;18(4):313–5.

91. Friel S. Occlusion. Observations on its development from infancy to old age. Int J Orthodontia, Oral Surg Radiography 1927;13(4):322–43.

92. Stuart CE. Good occlusion for natural teeth. J Prosthet Dent 1964;14(4):716–24.

93. Palla S. The interface of occlusion as a reflection of conflicts within prosthodontics. Int J Prosthodont 2005;18(4):304–6.

94. Mohl N. Diagnostic rationale: an overview. A textbook of occlusion 1988;179–84.

95. Celenza FV. The theory and clinical management of centric positions: I. Centric occlusion. Int J Periodontics Restorative Dent 1984;4(1):8–26.

96. Lux LH, Thompson GA, Waliszewski KJ, et al. Comparison of the Kois Dento-Facial Analyzer System with an earbow for mounting a maxillary cast. J Prosthet Dent 2015;114(3):432–9.

97. Seligman DA, Pullinger AG. The role of functional occlusal relationships in temporomandibular disorders: a review. J Craniomandib Disord 1991;5(4):265–79.

98. Gesch D, Bernhardt O, Mack F, et al. Association of malocclusion and functional occlusion with subjective symptoms of TMD in adults: results of the Study of Health in Pomerania (SHIP). Angle Orthod 2005;75(2):183–90.

99. Garrigós-Pedrón M, Elizagaray-García I, Domínguez-Gordillo AA, et al. Temporomandibular disorders: improving outcomes using a multidisciplinary approach. J Multidiscip Healthc 2019;12:733–47.

100. Greene CS, Obrez A. Treating temporomandibular disorders with permanent mandibular repositioning: is it medically necessary? Oral Surg Oral Med Oral Pathol Oral Radiol 2015;119(5):489–98.

101. Manfredini D, Perinetti G, Stellini E, et al. Prevalence of static and dynamic dental malocclusion features in subgroups of temporomandibular disorder patients: Implications for the epidemiology of the TMD-occlusion association. Quintessence Int 2015;46(4):341–9.

102. Yatani H, Minakuchi H, Matsuka Y, et al. The long-term effect of occlusal therapy on self-administered treatment outcomes of TMD. J Orofac Pain 1998;12(1):75–88.

103. Tsukiyama Y, Baba K, Clark GT. An evidence-based assessment of occlusal adjustment as a treatment for temporomandibular disorders. J Prosthet Dent 2001;86(1):57–66.

104. Fujii T. The relationship between the occlusal interference side and the symptomatic side in temporomandibular disorders. J Oral Rehabil 2003;30(3):295–300.

105. Chiappe G, Fantoni F, Landi N, et al. Clinical value of 12 occlusal features for the prediction of disc displacement with reduction (RDC/TMD Axis I group IIa). J Oral Rehabil 2009;36(5):322–9.

106. De Boever JA, Carlsson GE, Klineberg IJ. Need for occlusal therapy and prosthodontic treatment in the management of temporomandibular disorders. Part I. Occlusal interferences and occlusal adjustment. J Oral Rehabil 2000;27(5):367–79.

107. Report of the president's conference on the examination, diagnosis, and management of temporomandibular disorders. J Am Dent Assoc 1983;106(1):75–7.

108. Dixon DC. Diagnostic imaging of the temporomandibular joint. Dent Clin North Am 1991;35(1):53–74.

109. Mohl ND, Dixon DC. Current status of diagnostic procedures for temporomandibular disorders. J Am Dent Assoc 1994;125(1):56–64.

110. Kandasamy S, Boeddinghaus R, Kruger E. Condylar position assessed by magnetic resonance imaging after various bite position registrations. Am J Orthod Dentofacial Orthop 2013;144(4):512–7.

111. Alexander SR, Moore RN, DuBois LM. Mandibular condyle position: comparison of articulator mountings and magnetic resonance imaging. Am J Orthod Dentofacial Orthop 1993;104(3):230–9.
112. Rinchuse DJ, Kandasamy S. Articulators in orthodontics: an evidence-based perspective. Am J Orthod Dentofacial Orthop 2006;129(2):299–308.
113. Yohn K. The face bow is irrelevant for making prostheses and planning orthognathic surgery. J Am Dent Assoc 2016;147(6):421–6.

Temporomandibular Disorders Within the Context of Sleep Disorders

Daniele Manfredini, DDS, PhD[a],*,
Davis C. Thomas, BDS, DDS, MSD, MSc Med, MSc[b,c],
Frank Lobbezoo, DDS, PhD[d]

KEYWORDS

- Temporomandibular disorders • Sleep disorders • Bruxism
- Obstructive sleep apnea • Gastroesophageal reflux

KEY POINTS

- Most studies on the association between temporomandibular disorders (TMDs) and sleep disorders focused on sleep bruxism (SB).
- In general, questionnaire studies reported an association between TMDs and SB, whereas instrumental studies did not replicate such findings, likely because of the criteria adopted to assess SB.
- All studies relying on polysomnography/SB criteria were actually reporting on the association between pain and the number of masseter muscle activations associated with sleep arousals. Thus, they were not assessing the full spectrum of bruxism activities unrelated with sleep arousals and/or under the electromyography threshold for being considered an SB event.
- Concerning the relationship between TMDs and gastroesophageal reflux disease, and between TMDs and obstructive sleep apnea, there is a paucity of information, but an interaction between the conditions seems to exist and be worthy of further exploration.
- Clinicians working with patients with orofacial pain are encouraged to assess these factors when managing patients with TMD. To do that, multispecialist teams should be created that include professionals with different expertise.

[a] Facial Pain Unit, Department of Biomedical Technologies, School of Dentistry, University of Siena, Viale Bracci c/o Policlinico Le Scotte, Siena 53100, Italy; [b] Rutgers School of Dental Medicine, 110 Bergen St, Newark, NJ 07103, USA; [c] Eastman Institute of Oral Health, Rochester, NY, USA; [d] Department of Orofacial Pain and Dysfunction, Academic Centre for Dentistry Amsterdam (ACTA), University of Amsterdam and Vrije Universiteit Amsterdam, Gustav Mahlerlaan 3004, 1081 LA Amsterdam, the Netherlands
* Corresponding author.
E-mail address: daniele.manfredini@unisi.it

Dent Clin N Am 67 (2023) 323–334
https://doi.org/10.1016/j.cden.2022.10.004
0011-8532/23/© 2022 Elsevier Inc. All rights reserved.

INTRODUCTION

Temporomandibular disorders (TMDs) is a generic term that embraces different conditions affecting the temporomandibular joints (TMJs), the jaw muscles, and their related structures.[1] Muscle and/or joint pain, joint sounds during mandibular movements, and functional limitations are among the main signs and symptoms for which individuals seek for medical consultations. Generations of dentists have been educated according to a paradigm based on the importance of diagnosing and correcting purported abnormalities of dental occlusion and TMJ condyle position to manage patients with TMDs.[2] Nonetheless, over the past 3 decades, evidence emerged that such factors play a minor role, if any, in the cause of TMDs.[3–5] Conversely, a growing body of information supports the need to assess patients with TMD within the framework of a biopsychosocial model[6,7]; this led to a paradigm change in the evaluation[8,9] and treatment of TMDs.[10] Central factors concerning the psychological sphere and neurologic issues have become major aspects to address in the clinical and research settings.[11,12]

Within these premises, the role of sleep bruxism (SB) as a detrimental factor for the stomatognathic structures and as a possible trigger for TMD symptoms has already been debated for several decades.[13] Inconsistent findings have often emerged from instrumental studies (ie, based on polysomnography and/or electromyography) on SB with respect to the frequent clinical observation that patients with TMDs often report bruxism.[14,15] The study of such relationship provides complex clinical and research challenges and is further complicated by the emerging knowledge on other sleep disorders that may be of interest for the dental practitioner. Obstructive sleep apnea (OSA) and gastroesophageal reflux disease (GERD) are 2 examples of conditions included in the so-called circle of dental sleep disorders, which embraces multiple interacting conditions that may have a relationship with orofacial pains.[16]

Considering these emerging insights, this paper provides an overview of the knowledge on the relationship between TMDs and the main sleep conditions and disorders of dental interest, namely, SB, sleep apnea, and GERD. The main focus is be on TMDs and SB, which is by far the most studied topic and for which a historical framework will also be provided. Current evidence will be then adopted as a starting point for discussion of the clinical implications and a possible outline of future researches.

History

The association between SB and TMDs has been addressed by several systematic literature reviews. In particular, a paper by Manfredini and Lobbezoo,[14] which was published a decade ago and built on an earlier review by Lobbezoo and Lavigne,[13] concluded that research findings are influenced by the strategy adopted to assess bruxism. That review was not specifically aimed to discuss SB and included papers on bruxism in general. However, interesting conclusions could be drawn. Importantly, a pattern emerged to point out that investigations adopting a self-reported approach to bruxism found an association with TMDs, which was not fully replicated by the few investigations adopting strategies to measure SB instrumentally (ie, electromyography [EMG], polysomnography [PSG]).

Such findings must be interpreted by taking into account for the historical perspective of the definition of bruxism. For dental practitioners, bruxism has always been considered the act of grinding the teeth while asleep, a habit that in the early 90s was associated with the presence of specific patterns of masseter muscle activity (ie, rhythmic masticatory muscles activity [RMMA]) occurring time-linked to sleep arousals.[17] Dedicated PSG/SB screening criteria were developed based on the count of RMMA events per hour of sleep[18,19]; this contributed to the broadly diffused idea that bruxism, being synonymous of teeth grinding, is correlated with tooth wear, which is something that the literature has failed to fully support.[20–22] In addition, the adoption of PSG/SB criteria to study the possible association between SB and pain failed to show any relevant clinical relationship.[23]

After 2010, knowledge in the bruxism field has progressively evolved, leading to a paradigm shift and definition changes. Based on emerging evidence that bruxism should be viewed as an umbrella term including different motor behaviors, in 2013, an expert consensus panel provided a definition that reflects the complexity of the activity spectrum (ie, teeth grinding, teeth clenching, mandible bracing, mandible thrusting) and specifies that bruxism may have different circadian manifestations, namely, not only during sleep but also wakefulness (ie, awake bruxism).[24] In 2018, a successive paper further clarified this distinction and provided 2 separate definitions for sleep and awake bruxism.[25] SB, which is the focus of this paper, was defined as a masticatory muscle activity that occurs during sleep, characterized as rhythmic (phasic) or nonrhythmic (tonic) and not as a movement disorder or sleep disorder in otherwise healthy individuals.[25]

Different instrumental and noninstrumental approaches have been suggested as possible strategies for the assessment of SB, without necessarily having an unquestionable standard of reference. The ongoing works to finalize a Standardized Tool for the Assessment of Bruxism (STAB) reflect this open-minded, nonhierarchical approach to bruxism evaluation.[26] Indeed, although PSG is the ideal strategy to evaluate SB correlates, the count of the events is just one of the many outcome variables that may be evaluated as far as the jaw-muscle activity is concerned. Because of the lack of information on the amount of muscle work and duration, PSG may not be the ideal approach to evaluate the relationship between SB and signs and symptoms of TMDs.[27] On the other hand, the self-reported (eg, interviews, questionnaires) and clinical (eg, tooth wear, shiny spots on restorations, linea alba, tongue scalloping) approaches for the assessment of SB, which still remain the most adopted assessment strategies in large-sample studies, have well-known limits of accuracy in the differential diagnosis between different circadian bruxism activities as well as with respect to other conditions.[28] Thus, it is not surprising that findings on the relationship between bruxism and TMDs have been recently reevaluated in a comprehensive scoping review by Manfredini and Lobbezoo.[15]

Current Evidence

Temporomandibular disorders and sleep bruxism
The same inconsistency found in previous reviews has also been observed in the updated review of 2021,[15] which is limited to SB and covered all published papers on the relationship with TMDs. It confirmed that an association with TMDs is generally found in studies relying on self-reported or clinically based SB evaluation and is not confirmed in studies using instrumental approaches to its assessment (ie, PSG, EMG).

Some of the weak points underlined in 2010 are still present in the literature produced during the past decade, thus not allowing a real progress in knowledge with respect to the previous conclusions. Among those, it was pointed out that several articles did not focus on the TMD–SB association as their primary outcome, as well as that the adoption of different study designs and inclusion criteria made any data meta-analysis attempts impossible. Most instrumental studies had a control group of individuals not fulfilling PSG criteria for SB. With respect to such studies, the questionnaire-based investigations have a lower level of specificity for SB, which results from the frequently adopted single-item self-report (eg, the Research Diagnostic

Criteria for TMD [RDC/TMD] question for SB: Have you been told, or do you notice that you grind your teeth or clench your jaw while sleeping at night? Yes/No).[8] Such an approach is a potential bias for the study of the bruxism-pain association, as patients might tend to associate orofacial pain on awakening to a bruxism activity at night. In addition to that, population-based surveys are hardly useful to discriminate between individuals with clinically relevant symptoms who seek treatment and subjects who are just reporting an ancillary finding.

Thus, almost 25 years after the review by Lobbezoo and Lavigne[13] and more than 10 years after the review by Manfredini and Lobbezoo,[14] the relationship between SB and TMDs remains a debated topic. The updated review of 2021[15] led to confirm previous conclusions that observed associations strongly depend on the assessment strategy for SB. Indeed, in general, questionnaire studies reported an association between TMDs and SB, whereas instrumental studies did not, and even tended to point out the inverse relationship.[29] The clinical implications of these findings and some suggestions for designing future researches will be discussed later in this manuscript.

Temporomandibular disorders and other sleep disorders: obstructive sleep apnea and gastroesophageal reflux disease

One of most consistent findings from investigations on SB and TMDs is that tooth wear is not related with TMDs.[14,15] Indeed, all papers based on tooth wear assessment did not support an association with TMDs,[30–32] with minor exceptions concerning the possible value of attrition to discriminate between different TMD diagnoses.[33] These results may be of interest for general dental practitioners, who often tend to overly rely on old concepts of an ideal vertical dimension of occlusion as a needed parameter for the absence of TMD symptoms.[34] On the other hand, they also assume importance for the central role of tooth wear as a possible sign of the many conditions belonging to the circle of dental sleep disorders.[35]

Tooth wear is a multifactorial condition that requires a comprehensive qualitative and quantitative approach to its differential diagnosis.[36] Its relationship with dental sleep disorders has been the focus of many speculations. For details, readers are referred to the comprehensive review by Wetselaar and colleagues.[35] In summary, the importance of researches on tooth wear within the narrative of this paper is that they have allowed spotlighting the complex interactions between the various sleep disorders—some of them may have a direct association, whereas for some others it can be indirect.[35] Among the various dental sleep disorders, OSA and GERD are discussed later.

Population-based studies suggest that 4% of men and 2% of women aged more than 50 years suffer from symptomatic OSA syndrome, which is associated with clinical, psychological, and social impairment and is currently viewed as a major risk factor for several medical disorders.[37,38] Both anatomic and neurologic factors are involved in the development of obstruction of the upper airway in OSA.[39–44]

Within the multifactorial picture of dental sleep disorders, evidence on a possible relationship between TMDs and OSA is insufficient.[45] Concerning the association between the 2 conditions, data are scarce and can be mainly drawn from investigations on public health. In general, findings support the presence of a higher prevalence of TMDs in patients with OSA.[46] Interestingly, a recent large-scale study found a 2.8 higher risk than a control group,[47] confirming previous findings from the OPPERA study, which reported that a high likelihood of OSA is associated with 3.6 higher odds of chronic TMDs[48]; this may confirm the possible influence of poor sleep on the onset of painful orofacial conditions.[49,50] Clinical researches focused also on the possible TMD-related side effects in case of prolonged use of mandibular advancement devices (MAD) designed to manage OSA.[51,52] A meta-analysis suggests that MADs do not carry the risk to worsen TMD symptoms, despite some cautionary statements concerning the possible onset of transient symptoms at the individual level, which are generally mild.[53] On the other hand, there are no studies on the potential therapeutic effectiveness of OSA treatment on TMDs. As a concluding remark, despite this fragmented evidence, it seems reasonable to suggest that TMD screening in individuals who are deemed to receive an MAD as well as a screening for OSA in individuals with TMD is recommendable.[54,55]

The prevalence of GERD is high in the Western world, ranging from 10% to 40% based on literature data.[56] The prevalence increases with age and body mass index, and men are more frequently affected than women. Regurgitation, heartburn, and retrosternal pain are the main symptoms. Mild symptoms can be considered physiologic when occurring after a meal without further complaints and during pregnancy. Reflux becomes pathologic as a result from a combination of esophageal motility, lower esophageal sphincter function, and gastric motility or emptying, which leads to the development of clinical complaints.[57] From an etiologic perspective, GERD is considered a multifactorial disease, with obesity, age, and trauma representing the main risk factors. Within the circle of dental sleep disorders, GERD has been the target of several speculations concerning its possible association with SB, even if most studies actually focused on the relationship with tooth wear as a marker of a possible indirect association between both conditions.

Concerning the relationship between TMDs and GERD, there is a paucity of information, even if an association between the 2 conditions seems to exist and be worthy of further exploration.[58,59] In the case of both OSA and GERD, the study of the relationship with TMDs is thus complicated by their possible role as SB triggers,[60–62] which suggests the need to design studies that take into account for the complexity of the clinical picture at the individual level. In addition to that, it can also be considered that a specific pathophysiological mechanism for each factor interaction is not necessarily likely to exist and that the poor sleep quality of individuals with OSA, GERD, and SB may even emerge as the most important contributing factor for the onset of TMDs, in line with current thinking that disrupted sleep is a risk factor for pain.[63]

DISCUSSION

The relationship between TMDs and sleep disorders of dental interest is multifaceted. Its study is complicated by the fact that all the conditions described in this paper are associated with each other and all are multifactorial conditions. For some disorders, this association can be direct, whereas for others the association can be indirect or both. The multifactorial nature of these conditions has also led to a variety of assessment tools that were proposed over the years, which makes comparison of the findings in the literature difficult.

This issue is best exemplified by the literature on TMDs and SB, which is also the most explored topic among the various sleep conditions. For years, PSG has been considered the standard of reference to assess SB.[18,64] Because PSG/SB investigations did not retrieve any consistent pattern of association with TMDs, these findings have generally been interpreted as a proof of the absence of any relationship between SB and pain[23]; this was also one of the main arguments that led the proposal of considering bruxism "just" a behavior.[65] In addition to that, the fact that self-reported approaches to SB assessment found an association with TMDs[66–68] has been considered by some as an indirect proof of the lack of validity of SB self-report.[69] Based on this assumption, the 2013 consensus suggested the adoption of a diagnostic grading that provided that self-reported strategies may at best lead to a possible bruxism diagnosis, that the addition of a clinical evaluation would enhance the grade to probable bruxism, and that, in the case of SB, only PSG might achieve a definite diagnosis.[24] More recently, some criticism to the PSG/SB criteria have progressively emerged due to several observations.

According to the pain adaptation model and its integration, a protective reduction in muscle activity should be likely expected in individuals with pain.[70–72] That is exactly what has been found in individuals with experimentally induced pain, which in general causes a reduction in SB activity.[29,73] Besides, currently adopted PSG software analyses only include a count of the EMG events over a certain amplitude with respect to maximum voluntary clenching or to baseline levels, thus representing just a partial glimpse of the bruxism picture.[74] Within this framework, all studies relying on PSG/SB criteria were actually reporting on the association between pain and the number of masseter muscle activations associated with sleep arousals, namely, the activity that was taken as the reference to define an SB event. Thus, they were not assessing the full spectrum of bruxism activities unrelated with sleep arousals and/or under the EMG threshold for being considered an SB event; this is not a suitable strategy to investigate for the association with clinical consequences, due to the lack of information on total muscle work and masticatory muscles time index.[15] In addition to that, it must be pointed out that nonpainful symptoms, such as fatigue, stiffness, and tiredness, may be equally important in the clinical setting as pain.[75–77] Considering these drawbacks, a shift toward a more comprehensive, nonstackable approach to bruxism assessment has been suggested in the 2018 consensus[25] and adopted as a working strategy to define the STAB.[26]

These considerations have important clinical implications for the design of future studies, also concerning the other sleep disorders. In the case of SB, a possible clinical hypothesis is that prolonged, tonic muscle contractions or, more in general, the total amount of muscle activity during sleep are the actual key factors to explain the potential consequences of bruxism from a musculoskeletal viewpoint. Strategies to measure the muscle work,[78] assess the Bruxism Time Index,[79] or add info on the interval duration between events[80] are just examples of possible approaches to refine in the near future. The importance of such findings has been confirmed by the report of an increased background sleep-time masseter muscle activity in patients with myofascial pain with respect to healthy controls.[81] Thus, until new algorithms and suggestions for the interpretation of the EMG signal and validated SB metrics emerge,[82,83] it can be recommended to not discard all findings that are drawn from patients' self-report as if they are biased.[84]

Measuring of muscle activity could also be an interesting strategy to get a better depiction of the relationship between TMDs and the other sleep disorders. Indeed, on one hand, poor sleep quality may be a predictor of a reduced pain threshold[85–87]; on the other hand, abnormal muscle activity resulting from disrupted sleep may also be a concurrent factor to explain the relationship with TMD symptoms. Currently, there are no data on this issue, but preliminary observations pointed out an interesting pattern of prolonged tonic masseter contraction in some individuals with OSA during apnea-free periods of sleep.[62]

In consideration of that, further improvement on the interactions between conditions included in the circle of dental sleep disorders will be achieved with the design of investigations that take into account for the multiple comorbidities between the various disorders. SB seems to be a key factor that is interconnected with TMDs as well as with OSA and GERD. Emerging evidence suggests that SB should not be viewed as a stand-alone disorder, but rather as a sign of one or more underlying conditions.[28]

Both OSA and GERD can be examples of underlying conditions and, as such, they cannot be underestimated as risk factors for TMDs. The ongoing project for a multidimensional system for the evaluation of bruxism (ie, the STAB) is indeed going into the direction of collecting as many data as possible before building up any other hierarchical model for bruxism assessment in replacement of the old model that provided PSG as the standard of reference.[26] Nonetheless, PSG is crucial to study sleep architecture and will remain an essential strategy to screen for other sleep disorders that may be comorbid with TMDs. In addition to that, recent proposals for revising sleep apnea metrics in favor of a more patient-report oriented evaluation are examples of how all fields of dental sleep medicine are converging toward the common goal of defining a better correlation between instrumental and noninstrumental findings.[88] This could further open up a new era in the sleep disorders literature, with strong influence on the future research agenda for any investigations on their possible clinical consequences, such as TMDs. A recent scoping review identified the target of future instrumental research, which should aim to phenotype SB for both quantitative (eg, bruxism time index, bruxism work index) and qualitative (eg, arousal-related events, isolated short-lasting events, elevated background activity, tonic prolonged activity) evaluation.[15] The adoption of similar approaches to study OSA and GERD will surely shed light into their interconnection with SB and TMDs, both for research and clinical purposes.

SUMMARY

The relationship of TMDs with sleep conditions of dental interest, and SB in particular, has been reviewed in this paper. It emerged that, although the topic of SB as a possible detrimental factor for the stomatognathic structures has been the most studied, evidence is growing that SB, OSA, and GERD, all belong to a circle of mutually interacting sleep disorders and conditions that, in turn, may be associated with TMDs. The pathophysiology of the cause-and-effect relationships, if existing, has to be elucidated yet. Nonetheless, clinicians working with patients with orofacial pain are encouraged to assess these factors when managing patients with TMD. To do that, multispecialist teams should be created that include professionals with different expertise.

CLINICAL PEARLS

TMDs are a group of conditions that may present a multitude of complex interactions with sleep disorders. SB has been for decades considered a sleep disorder itself, but recent evidence pointed out that it should be better conceptualized as a muscle activity that may be a harmless finding or a sign of an underlying condition. Clinicians must thus be aware of the fact that the management of patients with TMDs may require a thorough evaluation of the presence of bruxism or any sleep disorder of dental interest, such as OSA and GERD in particular.

DISCLOSURE

The authors declare they do not have any conflicts of interest.

REFERENCES

1. De Leeuw R, Klasser GD, editors. The american academy of orofacial pain. Orofacial pain: guidelines for assessment, diagnosis and management. Chicago: Quintessence Publishing; 2017.

2. Okeson JP. Evolution of occlusion and temporomandibular disorder in orthodontics: Past, present, and future. Am J Orthod Dentofacial Orthop 2015;147(5 Suppl):S216–23.

3. Manfredini D, Lombardo L, Siciliani G. Temporomandibular disorders and dental occlusion. A systematic review of association studies: end of an era? J Oral Rehabil 2017;44(11):908–23.

4. Manfredini D. Occlusal Equilibration for the Management of Temporomandibular Disorders. Oral Maxillofac Surg Clin North Am 2018;30(3):257–64.

5. Greene CS, Manfredini D. Treating Temporomandibular Disorders in the 21st Century: Can We Finally Eliminate the "Third Pathway. J Oral Facial Pain Headache 2020;34(3):206–16.

6. Dworkin SF, Massoth DL. Temporomandibular disorders and chronic pain: disease or illness? J Prosthet Dent 1994;72(1):29–38.

7. Suvinen TI, Reade PC, Hanes KR, et al. Temporomandibular disorder subtypes according to self-reported physical and psychosocial variables in female patients: a re-evaluation. J Oral Rehabil 2005;32(3):166–73.

8. Dworkin SF, LeResche L. Research diagnostic criteria for temporomandibular disorders: review, criteria, examinations and specifications, critique. J Craniomandib Disord 1992;6(4):301–55.

9. Schiffman E, Ohrbach R, Truelove E, et al. International RDC/TMD Consortium Network, International association for Dental Research; Orofacial Pain Special Interest Group, International Association for the Study of Pain. Diagnostic Criteria for Temporomandibular Disorders (DC/TMD) for Clinical and Research Applications: recommendations of the International RDC/TMD Consortium Network* and Orofacial Pain Special Interest Group†. J Oral Facial Pain Headache 2014; 28(1):6–27.

10. Greene CS. The etiology of temporomandibular disorders: implications for treatment. J Orofac Pain 2001;15(2):93–105, discussion 106-16.

11. Ren K, Dubner R. Central nervous system plasticity and persistent pain. J Orofac Pain 1999;13(3):155–63, discussion 164-71.

12. Sessle BJ. Mechanisms of oral somatosensory and motor functions and their clinical correlates. J Oral Rehabil 2006;33(4):243–61.

13. Lobbezoo F, Lavigne GJ. Do bruxism and temporomandibular disorders have a cause-and-effect relationship? J Orofac Pain 1997;11(1):15–23.

14. Manfredini D, Lobbezoo F. Relationship between bruxism and temporomandibular disorders: a systematic review of literature from 1998 to 2008. Oral Surg Oral Med Oral Pathol Oral Radiol Endod 2010;109:e26–50.

15. Manfredini D, Lobbezoo F. Sleep bruxism and temporomandibular disorders: A scoping review of the literature. J Dent 2021;111:103711.

16. Lobbezoo F, Lavigne GJ, Kato T, et al. The face of Dental Sleep Medicine in the 21st century. J Oral Rehabil 2020;47(12):1579–89.

17. Macaluso GM, Guerra P, Di Giovanni G, et al. Sleep bruxism is a disorder related to periodic arousals during sleep. J Dent Res 1998;77(4):565–73.

18. Lavigne GJ, Rompré PH, Montplaisir JY. Sleep bruxism: validity of clinical research diagnostic criteria in a controlled polysomnographic study. J Dent Res 1996;75:546–52.

19. Rompré PH, Daigle-Landry D, Guitard F, et al. Identification of a sleep bruxism subgroup with a higher risk of pain. J Dent Res 2007;86:837–42.

20. Abe S, Yamaguchi T, Rompré PH, et al. Tooth wear in young subjects: a discriminator between sleep bruxers and controls? Int J Prosthodont 2009;22(4):342–50.

21. Manfredini D, Lombardo L, Visentin A, et al. Correlation between sleep-time masseter muscle activity and tooth wear: an electromyographic study. J Oral Facial Pain Headache 2019;33(2):199–204.
22. Kapagiannidou D, Koutris M, Wetselaar P, et al. Association between polysomnographic parameters of sleep bruxism and attrition-type tooth wear. J Oral Rehabil 2021;48(6):687–91.
23. Raphael KG, Sirois DA, Janal MN, et al. Sleep bruxism and myofascial temporomandibular disorders: a laboratory-based polysomnographic investigation. J Am Dent Assoc 2012;143:1223–31.
24. Lobbezoo F, Ahlberg J, Glaros AG, et al. Bruxism defined and graded: an international consensus. J Oral Rehabil 2013;40(1):2–4.
25. Lobbezoo F, Ahlberg J, Raphael KG, et al. International consensus on the assessment of bruxism: Report of a work in progress. J Oral Rehabil 2018;45:837–44.
26. Manfredini D, Ahlberg J, Aarab G, et al. Towards a Standardized Tool for the Assessment of Bruxism (STAB)-Overview and general remarks of a multidimensional bruxism evaluation system. J Oral Rehabil 2020;47(5):549–56.
27. Manfredini D, Ahlberg J, Wetselaar P, et al. The bruxism construct: from cut-off points to a continuum spectrum. J Oral Rehabil 2019;46:991–7.
28. Manfredini D, De Laat A, Winocur E, et al. Why not stop looking at bruxism as a black/white condition? aetiology could be unrelated to clinical consequences. J Oral Rehabil 2016;43:799–801.
29. Muzalev K, Visscher CM, Koutris M, et al. Effect of experimental temporomandibular disorder pain on sleep bruxism: a pilot study in males. Clin Oral Investig 2020;24(1):103–11.
30. John MT, Frank H, Lobbezoo F, et al. No association between incisal tooth wear and temporomandibular disorders. J Prosthet Dent 2002;87:197–203.
31. Janal MN, Raphael KG, Klausner J, et al. The role of tooth-grinding in the maintenance of myofascial face pain: a test of alternate models. Pain Med 2007;8:486–96.
32. Schierz O, John MT, Schroeder E, et al. Association between anterior tooth wear and temporomandibular disorder pain in a German population. J Prosthet Dent 2007;97:305–9.
33. Seligman DA, Pullinger AG. Dental attrition models predicting temporomandibular joint disease or masticatory muscle pain versus asymptomatic controls. J Oral Rehabil 2006;33:789–99.
34. Moreno-Hay I, Okeson JP. Does altering the occlusal vertical dimension produce temporomandibular disorders? A literature review. J Oral Rehabil 2015;42(11):875–82.
35. Wetselaar P, Manfredini D, Ahlberg J, et al. Associations between tooth wear and dental sleep disorders: a narrative overview. J Oral Rehabil 2019;46(8):765–75.
36. Wetselaar P, Lobbezoo F. The tooth wear evaluation system: a modular clinical guideline for the diagnosis and management planning of worn dentitions. J Oral Rehabil 2016;43(1):69–80.
37. Strollo PJ Jr, Rogers RM. Obstructive sleep apnea. N Engl J Med 1996;334:99–104.
38. Benjafield AV, Ayas NT, Eastwood PR, et al. Estimation of the global prevalence and burden of obstructive sleep apnoea: a literature-based analysis. Lancet Respir Med 2019;7(8):687–98.
39. Marchese-Ragona R, Vianello A, Restivo DA, et al. Sleep-related adductor laryngeal dystonia causing sleep apnea: a sleep-related breathing disorder

diagnosed with sleep endoscopy and treated with botulinum toxin. Laryngoscope 2013;123(6):1560–3.

40. Marchese-Ragona R, Manfredini D, Mion M, et al. Oral appliances for the treatment of obstructive sleep apnea in patients with low C-PAP compliance: a long-term case series. Cranio 2014;32(4):254–9.
41. Guarda-Nardini L, Manfredini D, Mion M, et al. Anatomically based outcome predictors of treatment for obstructive sleep apnea with intraoral splint devices: a systematic review of cephalometric studies. J Clin Sleep Med 2015;11(11):1327–34.
42. Chen H, Aarab G, de Ruiter MH, et al. Three-dimensional imaging of the upper airway anatomy in obstructive sleep apnea: a systematic review. Sleep Med 2016;21:19–27.
43. Gottlieb DJ, Punjabi NM. Diagnosis and management of obstructive sleep apnea: a review. JAMA 2020;23:1389–400.
44. Lobbezoo F, de Vries N, de Lange J, et al. A further introduction to dental sleep medicine. Nat Sci Sleep 2020;12:1173–9.
45. Al-Jewair T, Shibeika D, Ohrbach R. Temporomandibular Disorders and Their Association with Sleep Disorders in Adults: A Systematic Review. J Oral Facial Pain Headache 2021;35(1):41–53.
46. Alessandri-Bonetti A, Scarano E, Fiorita A, et al. Prevalence of signs and symptoms of temporo-mandibular disorder in patients with sleep apnea. Sleep Breath 2021;25(4):2001–6.
47. Wu JH, Lee KT, Kuo CY, et al. The association between temporomandibular disorder and sleep apnea-a nationwide population-based cohort study. Int J Environ Res Public Health 2020;17(17):6311.
48. Sanders AE, Essick GK, Fillingim R, et al. Sleep apnea symptoms and risk of temporomandibular disorder: OPPERA cohort. J Dent Res 2013;92(7 Suppl):70S–7S.
49. Almoznino G, Benoliel R, Sharav Y, et al. Sleep disorders and chronic craniofacial pain: Characteristics and management possibilities. Sleep Med Rev 2017;33:39–50.
50. Klasser GD, Almoznino G, Fortuna G. Sleep and orofacial pain. Dent Clin North Am 2018;62(4):629–56.
51. Doff MH, Veldhuis SK, Hoekema A, et al. Long-term oral appliance therapy in obstructive sleep apnea syndrome: a controlled study on temporomandibular side effects. Clin Oral Investig 2012;16(3):689–97.
52. Nikolopoulou M, Aarab G, Ahlberg J, et al. Oral appliance therapy versus nasal continuous positive airway pressure in obstructive sleep apnea: A randomized, placebo-controlled trial on temporomandibular side-effects. Clin Exp Dent Res 2020;6(4):400–6.
53. Alessandri-Bonetti A, Bortolotti F, Moreno-Hay I, et al. Effects of mandibular advancement device for obstructive sleep apnea on temporomandibular disorders: A systematic review and meta-analysis. Sleep Med Rev 2019;48:101211.
54. Merrill RL. Temporomandibular disorder pain and dental treatment of obstructive sleep apnea. Dent Clin North Am 2012;56(2):415–31.
55. Mehta NR, Correa LP. Oral Appliance Therapy and Temporomandibular Disorders. Sleep Med Clin 2018;13(4):513–9.
56. Mikami DJ, Murayama KM. Physiology and pathogenesis of gastroesophageal reflux disease. Surg Clin North Am 2015;95(3):515–25.
57. Fock KM, Poh CH. Gastroesophageal reflux disease. J Gastroenterol 2010;45(8):808–15.

58. Gharaibeh TM, Jadallah K, Jadayel FA. Prevalence of temporomandibular disorders in patients with gastroesophageal reflux disease: a case-controlled study. J Oral Maxillofac Surg 2010;68(7):1560–4.

59. Li Y, Fang M, Niu L, et al. Associations among gastroesophageal reflux disease, mental disorders, sleep and chronic temporomandibular disorder: a case-control study. CMAJ 2019;191(33):E909–15.

60. Ohmure H, Oikawa K, Kanematsu K, et al. Influence of experimental esophageal acidification on sleep bruxism: a randomized trial. J Dent Res 2011;90(5):665–71.

61. Manfredini D, Guarda-Nardini L, Marchese-Ragona R, et al. Theories on possible temporal relationships between sleep bruxism and obstructive sleep apnea events. An Expert Opinion Sleep Breath 2015;19:1459–65.

62. Colonna A, Cerritelli L, Lombardo L, et al. Temporal relationship between sleeptime masseter muscle activity and apnea-hypopnea events: A pilot study. J Oral Rehabil 2022;49(1):47–53.

63. Cohen SP, Vase L, Hooten WM. Chronic pain: an update on burden, best practices, and new advances. Lancet 2021;397(10289):2082–97.

64. Lavigne GJ, Khoury S, Abe S, et al. Bruxism physiology and pathology: an overview for clinicians. J Oral Rehabil 2008;35(7):476–94.

65. Raphael KG, Santiago V, Lobbezoo F. Is bruxism a disorder or a behavior? Rethinking the international consensus on defining and grading of bruxism. J Oral Rehabil 2016;43:791–8.

66. Huang GJ, Leresche L, Critchlow CW, et al. Risk factors for diagnostic subgroups of painful temporomandibular disorders (TMD). J Dent Res 2002;81:284–8.

67. Manfredini D, Cantini E, Romagnoli M, et al. Prevalence of bruxism in patients with different research diagnostic criteria for temporomandibular disorders (RDC/TMD) diagnoses. Cranio 2003;21(4):279–85.

68. Manfredini D, Winocur E, Guarda-Nardini L, et al. Self-reported bruxism and temporomandibular disorders: findings from two specialised centres. J Oral Rehabil 2012;39(5):319–25.

69. Raphael KG, Janal MN, Sirois DA, et al. Validity of self-reported sleep bruxism among myofascial temporomandibular disorder patients and controls. J Oral Rehabil 2015;42(10):751–8.

70. Lund JP, Donga R, Widmer CG, et al. The pain-adaptation model: a discussion of the relationship between chronic musculoskeletal pain and motor activity. Can J Physiol Pharmacol 1991;69:683–94.

71. Murray GM, Peck CC. Orofacial pain and jaw muscle activity: a new model. J Orofac Pain 2007;21:263–78.

72. Manfredini D, Cocilovo F, Stellini E, et al. Surface electromyography findings in unilateral myofascial pain patients: comparison of painful vs. non painful sides. Pain Med 2013;14(12):1848–53.

73. Santiago V, Raphael K. Absence of joint pain identifies high levels of sleep masticatory muscle activity in myofascial temporomandibular disorder. J Oral Rehabil 2019;46(12):1161–9.

74. Manfredini D, Ahlberg J, Lobbezoo F. Bruxism definition: Past, present, and future - What should a prosthodontist know? J Prosthet Dent 2021;S0022-3913(21): 00074–83.

75. Slade GD, Ohrbach R, Greenspan JD, et al. Painful Temporomandibular Disorder: Decade of Discovery from OPPERA Studies. J Dent Res 2016;95(10): 1084–92.

76. Thymi M, Shimada A, Lobbezoo F, et al. Clinical jaw-muscle symptoms in a group of probable sleep bruxers. J Dent 2019;85:81–7.

77. Shimada A, Castrillon EE, Svensson P. Revisited relationships between probable sleep bruxism and clinical muscle symptoms. J Dent 2019;82:85–90. https://doi. org/10.1016/j.jdent.2019.01.013. Epub 2019 Feb 1. PMID: 30716450.
78. Manfredini D, Fabbri A, Peretta R, et al. Influence of psychological symptoms on home-recorded sleep-time masticatory muscle activity in healthy subjects. J Oral Rehabil 2011;38(12):902–11.
79. Van der Zaag J, Lobbezoo F, Visscher CM, et al. Time-variant nature of sleep bruxism outcome variables using ambulatory polysomnography: implications for recognition and therapy evaluation. J Oral Rehabil 2008;35:577–84.
80. Muzalev K, Lobbezoo F, Janal MN, et al. Interepisode Sleep Bruxism Intervals and Myofascial Face Pain. Sleep 2017;40(8):zsx078.
81. Raphael KG, Janal MN, Sirois DA, et al. Masticatory muscle sleep background electromyographic activity is elevated in myofascial temporomandibular disorder patients. J Oral Rehabil 2013;40(12):883–91.
82. Lavigne G, Kato T, Herrero Babiloni A, et al. Research routes on improved sleep bruxism metrics: Toward a standardised approach. J Sleep Res 2021;30(5): e13320.
83. Thymi M, Lobbezoo F, Aarab G, et al. Signal acquisition and analysis of ambulatory electromyographic recordings for the assessment of sleep bruxism: a scoping review. J Oral Rehabil 2021;48(7):846–71.
84. Manfredini D, Colonna A, Bracci A, et al. Bruxism: a summary of current knowledge on aetiology, assessment, and management. Oral Surg 2020;13:358–70.
85. Engstrøm M, Hagen K, Bjørk M, et al. Sleep quality, arousal and pain thresholds in tension-type headache: a blinded controlled polysomnographic study. Cephalalgia 2014;34(6):455–63.
86. Larson RA, Carter JR. Total sleep deprivation and pain perception during cold noxious stimuli in humans. Scand J Pain 2016;13:12–6.
87. Iacovides S, George K, Kamerman P, et al. Sleep fragmentation hypersensitizes healthy young women to deep and superficial experimental pain. J Pain 2017; 18(7):844–54.
88. Pevernagie DA, Gnidovec-Strazisar B, Grote L, et al. On the rise and fall of the apnea-hypopnea index: a historical review and critical appraisal. J Sleep Res 2020;29(4):e13066.

Myofascial Temporomandibular Disorders at a Turning Point
Pragmatic or Evidence-Based Management?

Julyana Gomes Zagury, DMD, MSD,
Sowmya Ananthan, BDS, DMD, MSD, Samuel Y.P. Quek, DMD, MPH*,
Gayathri Subramanian, BDS, PhD, DMD

KEYWORDS

- Myofascial orofacial pain • Masticatory myofascial temporomandibular disorders
- Chronic pain • Evidence-based approach • Diagnosis • Management

KEY POINTS

- Although several theories have been raised, the true etiopathogenesis of masticatory myofascial temporomandibular disorders (mTMD) remains unknown.
- Diagnosis is merely centered on establishing "familiar pain" on palpating or mobilizing masticatory myofascial tissue.
- This results in subjective assessments of both the severity of the disease and of ascertaining treatment response.
- No rigorous means exists to compare treatment efficacy or to assign a given treatment option. Inadequate management may perpetuate pain, risking reliance on opioids.
- Hence, a pragmatic approach to mTMD is suboptimal; emerging technologies show promise in identifying biomarkers and objectively assessing myofascial tissue in health and disease.

INTRODUCTION

Approximately a third of the world's population may experience some form of chronic pain.[1,2] Chronic pain tends to impact women, individuals from lower socioeconomic and/or rural backgrounds, and even veterans more so than others, and a higher prevalence of both chronic pain in general, as well as high-impact chronic pain, are encountered in these subgroups.[1] An estimated 11 to 12 million US adults experienced chronic pain in and around the region of the temporomandibular joint, which

Department of Diagnostic Sciences, Rutgers School of Dental Medicine, 110 Bergen Street, Newark, NJ, USA
* Corresponding author.
E-mail address: queksa@sdm.rutgers.edu

could be related to temporomandibular disorders (TMD).[3] It is notable that the prevalence of any high-impact chronic pain is approximately fourfold in patients with orofacial symptoms.[3] Annual TMD-related health care costs are estimated to be around $4 billion each year, signifying its profound impact.[4,5]

This narrative review and perspective focuses on masticatory myofascial/myogenous temporomandibular disorders (henceforth referred to as myofascial temporomandibular disorders [mTMD] in this article), the most prevalent subtype of TMDs and affects approximately 5 million people in the United States.[3,6,7]

Diagnosis, Assessment, and Management of Myofascial Temporomandibular Disorders

mTMD is diagnosed using the duplication of "familiar pain" on palpation of the myofascial tissue, commonly over the masseter and temporalis muscles or with maximum assisted or unassisted mouth opening movement(s) (**Table 1**).[8] A recent update to the classification of orofacial pain updated the classification of myofascial orofacial pain (analogous to mTMD) into primary orofacial pain as well as secondary, attributable to tendonitis, myositis, and muscle spasm as shown by clinical examination. This was further subdivided based on chronicity and frequency of pain (**Box 1**).[9] Unlike temporomandibular joint disorders (TMJ disorders), the use of diagnostic testing beyond clinical examination, for example, using computed tomography (CT), conebeam CT (CBCT) or MRI is mostly non-contributory toward the diagnosis of mTMD.[10]

Chronic pain, in general, is multifactorial with a reciprocal or bidirectional emotional and psychosocial impact. Clinical examination of Axis I and Axis II features is critical to a comprehensive assessment of TMDs.[8,11] Further, emerging insight implicates central mechanisms to the perpetuation and perception of chronic pain (nociplastic pain), although the extent of this impact may vary and is complex to assess.[12–14] It is not surprising that the assessment and management of mTMD remains challenging.

An essential consideration in the assessment and management of mTMD is that several theories have been proposed to explain the etiopathogenesis of mTMD; however, similar to other chronic pain phenomena, these theories are not rigorously validated. As a consequence, a variety of empirical strategies for the management of mTMD exist in clinical use that are not well-validated as well. This lack of clarity in the pathogenesis of mTMD is a bottleneck to the optimal assessment and management of mTMD. The key consequences and implications of the current status quo are summarized in the sections below.

Common Modalities of Management

Currently, mTMD is mostly managed in a conservative manner (approaches listed in **Table 2**), following the biopsychosocial model. Noninvasive strategies include counseling, the use of occlusal appliances, acupuncture, physical therapy, low-level laser therapy, and pharmacologic management, among others. More invasive treatment modalities include local anesthetics in the context of trigger point injections, peripheral nerve blocks, systemic medications, and neuromodulation and have been used to manage persistent mTMD, which is refractory to conservative treatment.

Counseling involves a range of interventions from patient education through selfcare to more targeted and specific cognitive-behavioral therapy (CBT). CBT is a time-limited, problem-focused psychotherapy applicable to a wide range of conditions ranging from depression, anxiety disorder, chronic pain, and substance abuse to eating disorders.[15] In addition to education on TMD, self-care advocacy, and setting patient expectations, CBT is focused on reducing specific maladaptive behavior and augmenting adaptive patient cognition and behavior. Often, counseling

Table 1
Validated axis I pain-related temporomandibular disorder diagnoses

Disorder	History	Examination Findings
Myalgia • Sens: 90% • Spec: 99%	Pain in a masticatory structure modified by jaw movement, function, or parafunction	Report of familiar pain in temporalis or masseter muscle(s) with: 1. Palpation of these muscles, or 2. Maximum unassisted or assisted opening movement(s). Note: Assessment of other masticatory muscles may be indicated in some clinical situations.
Myofascial pain with referral • Sens: 86% • Spec: 98%	Same as for myalgia	1. Report of familiar pain with palpation of the temporalis or masseter muscle(s) and 2. Report of pain at a site beyond the boundary of the muscle being palpate (eg, referral to a tooth)

Reproduced in part, from Schiffman E, Ohrbach R, Truelove E, et al. Diagnostic Criteria for Tempo-romandibular Disorders (DC/TMD) for Clinical and Research Applications: recommendations of the International RDC/TMD Consortium Network* and Orofacial Pain Special Interest Groupdagger. *J Oral Facial Pain Headache.* 2014;28(1):6-27.

is delivered in conjunction with other intervention(s). Counseling strategies have shown benefits in the context of both acute and chronic pain.[16]

Oral appliances have been the mainstay of mTMD management.[17] Multiple designs have been used and described in the literature. It seems that a full-coverage hard acrylic appliance that rests on either maxillary or mandibular arches, with bilateral centric contacts against the opposite arch, may have the most stable performance, with minimal chances for occlusal changes. Patient compliance and regular follow-up are essential for eliciting clinical benefit.[18]

Acupuncture involves the insertion of multiple thin, solid needles in specific points termed "acupoints," by trained professionals, in a series of visits. Multiple methods have been advocated for improving pain-limited mouth opening as well as the quality of life.[19]

Physical therapy for mTMD is centered on tissue manipulation, involving the soft tissues and joints of the head and neck, again involving multiple sessions. Desired outcomes include relief of muscle spasms and "local adhesions," with improved local circulation, resulting in improved range of motion and reduced pain.[20,21]

Photobiomodulation therapy with low-level laser therapy is believed to enhance healing with regenerative potential,[22] with evidence for improved functional outcomes, minimal adverse effects, and good patient acceptance.[23] It should, however, be noted that there is a high variability in laser type, frequency of use, exposure time, and duration of treatment.

Trigger point injection refers to the technique of administering a local anesthetic into an identifiable trigger point in a taut band of skeletal muscle.[24] Trigger point injections have consistently shown pain alleviation and improvement in mouth opening for at least 6 months.[25] Technique sensitivity and the accurate diagnosis, localization, and

> **Box 1**
> **International Classification of Pain (ICOP) classification of myofascial orofacial pain**
>
> Myofascial orofacial pain
> - Primary myofascial orofacial pain
>   - Acute primary myofascial orofacial pain
>   - Chronic primary myofascial orofacial pain
> - Secondary myofascial orofacial pain
>   - Myofascial orofacial pain attributed to tendonitis
>   - Myofascial orofacial pain attributed to myositis
>   - Myofascial orofacial pain attributed to muscle spasm
>
> Classification of chronic primary myofascial orofacial pain based on frequency
> - Infrequent (onset > 3 months ago, occurring on <1 d/mo of each episode at least 30 min, for at least 2 h in a day)
> - Frequent (onset > 3 months ago, occurring 1–14 days a month, >12 days but <180 d/y)
> - Highly frequent (occurring on >15 d/mo on average for >3 months (>180 d/y))
>
> (Adapted from International Classification of Orofacial Pain, 1st edition (ICOP). Cephalalgia. 2020;40(2):129–221.)

manipulation of the trigger point for medication delivery are essential for a predictable response. In contrast, dry needling involves the insertion of solid needles into trigger points, tendons, ligaments, and scar tissue. This modality is believed to reduce peripheral pain and sensitization.[26,27]

The use of peripheral nerve blocks for the management of mTMD is relatively new, with early evidence of efficacy, though the use of peripheral nerve blocks in the general management of myofascial pain itself is not new.[28–31] The temporomassteric nerve block (TNMB aka the Twin block) is a peripheral regional nerve block that targets the innervation to the temporalis and masseter muscles.[32–34]

Several pharmacologic interventions are commonplace in mTMD management, though with low-rigor validation.[35] They range from nonsteroidal anti-inflammatory drugs (NSAIDs) (primarily in the context of short-term management of acute painful episodes), to tricyclic antidepressants (TCA), favored due to relative safety profile and placative impact on sleep and mood disorders (though adverse events have been noted with amitryptiline more often than nortryptyline), to skeletal muscle relaxants, namely benzodiazepines such as clonazepam (addiction potential is a caution) and less often, cyclobenzaprine. Pain alleviation with opioids has no mechanistic potential yet has a high risk for dependence. Neuromodulation strategies used in chronic pain, in general, include interventions such as transcutaneous electrical nerve stimulation (TENS) and other more invasive direct nerve stimulation (ranging from peripheral, dorsal root ganglion, spinal cord, to brain stimulation) are primarily explored in the context of failed therapies and are not rigorously validated.[36] Their use is primarily in the context of neuropathic pain and much less in myofascial pain.

It is not feasible to objectively determine the actual effect these treatment modalities have, and various combinations are often used simultaneously or over time. mTMD management is thus dictated by what we know, that is, a pragmatic approach driven by practical rather than theoretic considerations. It should be appreciated that how much we do not understand or comprehend mTMD, marginalizes us to a narrow fringe of focusing on pain mitigation as the only pragmatic treatment option available to intervene in mTMD. Chronic pain is the common denominator used in the diagnosis, assessment, and the therapeutic target in mTMD. The Diagnostic Criteria for Temporomandibular Disorders (DC/TMD) Criteria (see **Table 1**) are based on eliciting

Table 2	
Management modalities in myofascial temporomandibular disorders	
Conservative Treatment of mTMD	
Counseling	Patient education
	Self-performed exercises
	Parafunctional habit management/awareness
	Thermal compresses
	Physical activity
	Mindfulness
	Relaxation
	Cognitive behavioral therapy
	Psychosocial burden—self/professional assessment
Occlusal appliances	Multiple designs
Pharmacotherapy	Systemic
	NSAIDs
	Acetaminophen
	Muscle relaxants
	TCAs (tricyclic antidepressants)
	Opioids
	NMDA inhibitor
	Alpha agonists
	Others
	Topical
	NSAIDs
	Lidocaine
Physical/chiropractic therapy	Manual manipulation
	Exercises
Low-level laser therapy	Multiple variations
Therapeutic ultrasound	
Dry needling	
Trigger point injections	Ultrasound-guided or blinded
	multiple local anesthetics
Peripheral nerve block	Temporomasseteric nerve block
Acupuncture	Multiple modalities
Hypnosis	
Others	
Concomitant management of comorbidities (anxiety, depression, and other chronic pain conditions)	

"familiar," localized, or radiating pain on palpation of the musculoskeletal tissue or on its mobilization.[8] Although highly specific and sensitive for myalgia ("pain in muscle" from either muscular or fascial tissue, or both), the diagnostic accuracy of the DC/TMD criteria is lower for the subtypes. Thus, the diagnosis of "myalgia" is reliable, using elicited familiar pain as the diagnostic criterion. The pain response varies from individual to individual, making it an inappropriate tool for comparing the severity of mTMD in patients. In addition, using pain management interventions as a treatment only addresses the consequence of mTMD and not its etiology. Lastly, it is difficult to meaningfully distinguish between primary and secondary chronic myofascial orofacial pain, given that we still do not know the true mechanism/s of the disease process.[9] Only a low level of evidence exists for the validation of the current international classification of pain in this category, primarily relying on inter-rater variability and subjective assessments.[37]

Making a Case for Evidence-Based Management

Philosophically, an approach that is diametrically opposed to being pragmatic is an evidence-based approach. At this time, although the literature is rife with individual commentaries, case series, and even systematic reviews of individual interventions, high-quality evidence in the form of randomized assignment of treatment options to patients who have been objectively assessed at baseline and for treatment response, is unavailable.[20,38–46] Thus, evidence-based guidelines for the optimal management of mTMD are nonexistent. Ironically, between both approaches, pragmatic and evidence-based clinical decision-making, as the field stands today, neither approach can be judged superior as a result of inadequate data. This impasse results from several factors:

a. Lack of objective basis for treatment assignment: Choice of treatment in mTMD is often determined arbitrarily by the training/experience/skill set of the clinician-much like "if all you have is a hammer, everything looks like a nail." The dentist is not the only practitioner who evaluates and treats patients with mTMD. In a pragmatic clinical setting, because the skills required for different treatment options are often nonoverlapping, a true choice among treatment options, for example, tissue manipulation versus oral appliance versus acupuncture, may not exist. This may be the reason why high-quality interdisciplinary studies for rigorous comparison of interventions are lacking.
b. We cannot assess what we cannot/do not measure: The pathophysiological changes in myofascial tissue in mTMD remain unelucidated. As a result, there are no established tissue parameters that reflect disease severity or complexity. It is thus impossible to stratify or group mTMD patients according to any objective parameter that can be quantified. The only measurable parameter is pain.
c. Chronic pain is semiquantitative, subjective, and complex: Pain in chronic pain conditions is difficult to assess. The psychosocial and emotional burden of chronic pain conditions can impact pain perception and interpretation.[47–49] Through observational studies of the natural course of chronic pain conditions, it is known that pain tends to vary over time.[50] This variability can confound interpretation of any response to intervention/s and thus complicate assessment. In addition, in conditions such as chronic lower back pain, pain intensity has been observed to level over time regardless of whether the intervention was surgical or not.[51]

The field is currently at its crossroads-it is accepted that the current management of mTMD is largely empirical and suboptimal.[49,52] The very nature of such a pragmatic approach to management precludes the accumulation of evidence, making it nearly impossible to create a broad foundation for a truly evidence-based approach to guide mTMD management. Unless we drastically change our approach in mTMD, we are unlikely to change this status quo.

The lack of an objective assessment and management of mTMD contributes to poorly managed chronic pain, potentially amplifying the psychosocial burden and reliance on opioid medications to palliate pain.[53] As long as the management of mTMD remains suboptimal and heavily focused on pain management; it will contribute to the current prescription opioid crisis; the burden of unmitigated chronic pain perpetuates the risk of substance use disorder.

It is also essential to address the possibility that using established chronic pain to diagnose mTMD may delay its diagnosis and allow the underlying disease mechanism/s to perpetuate, feeding into its chronicity. Investigating underlying mechanisms may enable an earlier window of opportunity to detect and mitigate the problem at an earlier stage. Identifying specific myofascial tissue parameter/s that are deranged in mTMD will enable us to assess disease severity objectively instead of relying on pain severity as a surrogate. This will further enable the design, conduct, and evaluation of therapeutic interventions in a rigorous manner, greatly facilitating the progress of evidence-based research.

Lastly, in addition to mTMD, myofascial pain impacts many other severe and chronic pain conditions, such as chronic lower back pain, neck and shoulder pain, and headache. Thus, progress in elucidating the mechanistic basis for mTMD can enhance our understanding of these related clinical phenomena as well. Thus, the argument for shifting the current paradigm of management of mTMD is compelling and timely. The field of mTMD management is primed for a strategic shift toward objective quantitative assessment and characterization of normal myofascial tissues to distinguish features unique to mTMD.

As the first step in this direction, we need to acknowledge what we do not know, and that can be accomplished only after we gauge all that is "known" and judge if it is based on credible research that translates to actual clinical presentations.

The Etiopathogenesis of Myofascial Temporomandibular Disorders Has Not Been Elucidated

The etiopathogenesis of acute mTMD pain (summarized schematically in **Fig. 1**) is typically associated with traumatic injury, infection, or ultrastructural muscle damage resulting from unaccustomed eccentric and concentric contractions (in delayed onset muscle soreness), or high demand of skeletal muscle load by sustained low-level contraction or dynamic repetitive contraction.[54] All lead to acute mTMD due to an associated local inflammation, local metabolite accumulation, and muscle damage, resulting in muscle nociception sensitization and potential central sensitization, in addition to maintenance of muscle contraction through a vicious cycle. In addition, there is a potentially relevant role of deep fascia that intimately surrounds the muscle.[55,56]

Most acute mTMD are self-limiting or resolve once the infection or inflammation is properly addressed. The challenge rests on the etiopathogenesis of persistent or recurrent chronic mTMD, which has been based mainly on speculations and assumptions. In fact, the relationship between sustained muscle overload, such as clenching or bruxism, and mTMD is still controversial.[57,58] Experimental studies have shown that not all individuals may develop pain following clenching or eccentric, concentric jaw closing exercises, and such parafunctional habit alone is not able to result in chronic myofascial pain.[58,59] Interestingly, parafunctional habits are considered one of the risk factors for the development of myogenous TMD, and it might emerge from the emotional motor system under a raised psychological burden.[48,57,60] In addition, the presence of local algogenic substances in the muscles differs through different stages of mTMD pain, not necessarily with direct association to chronic mTMD pain intensity or tenderness.[61]

Peripheral and central sensitization (suggestive of nociplastic pain, with varying levels of amplified processing and/or reduced inhibition of pain nociception at multiple levels in the nervous system)[12,14] may play a role in the maintenance or perpetuation of mTMD pain. However, the relative contribution between these and local factors may be tipped toward predominantly local factors in myalgia/myofascial pain without referral versus a more dominant role of the central nervous system (CNS) in myofascial pain with a referral.[13] In addition, the interchange between muscle nociception and both emotion and psychosocial burden (psychological input), motor function, autonomic nervous system, and sleep, as well as the neuroimmune interplay, might be involved in the pathophysiology of chronic musculoskeletal pain. Comorbidities associated with a subgroup of chronic masticatory and cervical muscle pain, such as sleep

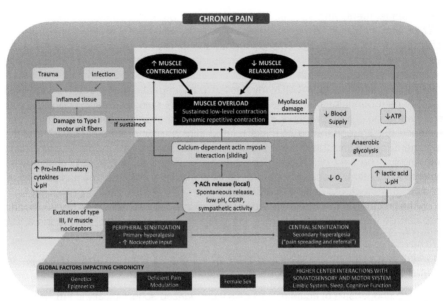

Fig. 1. Theories of mTMD pathophysiology. High muscle demand may yield in a local reduction of capillary flow (ischemia), low oxygen supply (hypoxia), and energy crisis (lack of ATP), resulting in tissue damage.[79–81] With low oxygen availability, the source of energy (ATP) changes from aerobic to anaerobic glycolysis, which produces less ATP and more lactic acid. The sustained contraction may delay the elimination of lactic acid from the tissue. Thus, there is a local decrease in ATP availability and an increase in acidity (low pH).[79] Although the lack of ATP interferes with relaxation and accumulates intracellular calcium, low pH stimulates muscle nociceptors,[82] which in turn release neuropeptides (eg, CGRP), further sensitizing the muscle nociceptor. The role of low pH and ATP in muscle nociceptor pain has been associated with various muscle pain conditions. Low pH (increased proton) and CGRP released from nociceptors may also intensify Ach action. They act in different modes, either by inhibiting the action of acetylcholinesterase at the synaptic cleft increasing the efficacy of Ach (low pH and CGRP) or by promoting upregulation of acetylcholine receptors (CGRP). More acetylcholine at the motor endplate maintains muscle contraction.

disturbances, altered cognitive function, or generalized pain, suggest pain processing malfunctioning at the level of the CNS.[62,63] Genetics and epigenetics also seem to contribute significantly to the development and maintenance of chronic pain.[64]

A typical characteristic of mTMD is a higher prevalence of females affected. Studies have shown that in acute mTMD, there is no statistically significant difference between males and females.[54,65] However, female predominance is observed in chronic TMD. There is evidence of differences between genders regarding trigeminal nociceptive pathway and central sensitization that might partially explain such differences.

Emerging Tools to Assess Myofascial Temporomandibular Disorders, and to Measure Myofascial Tissue Health and Function

Recent studies have been looking into potential biomarkers for chronic muscle pain.[63] A combination of biomarkers may be preferable over single biomarkers due to the variability of clinical conditions, multiple pain presentations, and comorbidities.[63,66] The biomarkers may include molecular, neuroimaging, neurosensory/motor (eg, quantitative sensory testing), genetic/epigenetic, or biochemical.[63,67] Zinc, serotonin, glutamate, lactate, pyruvate, dopamine, cytokines, growth factors, neuropeptides, catecholamines, matrix metalloproteinases, and oxidative stress markers have been suggested as potential bio-markers, but some are still controversial and more research is required.[68] The advantage of assessments such as serum biomarker(s), compared with tissue-specific assays, may be that given the unclear etiopathogenesis, biomarkers in circulation can potentially reflect a diseased state, regardless of tissue of origin.

Technological resources, even though in their infancy in their utilization on mTMD, may assist in expanding our understanding of mTMD physiology and pathophysi-ology. They include salivary markers detectors,[69] ultrasound that may guide more precisely target regions to be treated and assess local changes, such as edema;[70] functional brain MRI (fMRI), and specific MRI techniques, such as diffusion tensor imaging (DTI), may assess functional abnormalities at CNS involved in mTMD, whereas DTI may also assess lateral pterygoid muscle function,[71–74] magnetization transfer contrast imaging for detection of intramuscular edema or local ischemia,[74] and intramuscular microdialysis for detection of local molecular changes.[61,75–78]

The way forward

We have an obligation to aim for well-designed studies to apply the current knowledge of masticatory myofascial physiology and pathophysiology, including peripheral and central adaptation competence, and expand further in the search for a better under-standing of the condition and for potential biomarkers that may serve as objective measures. This will greatly facilitate our ability to assess the effectiveness of treatment modalities. Gathering such evidence may be the true pragmatic approach to optimally diagnosing and managing mTMD.

CLINICS CARE POINTS

- Temporomandibular disorder (mTMD) etiopathogenesis has not been fully elucidated; theories for mTMD development have not been validated.

- mTMD seems to have both nociceptive and nociplastic (pain processing and perception) components.

- The diagnosis of "myalgia" per the current the Diagnostic Criteria for Temporomandibular Disorders criteria has higher diagnostic accuracy than further subtypes.

- Currently, mTMD diagnosis and management are both centered on a subjective, and hence variable assessment of pain.

- A variety of treatment options exist for the management of mTMD; these are primarily based on the biopsychosocial model. It is not feasible to objectively compare interventions due to incomplete assessment of disease severity at baseline and response to treatment beyond the subjective assessment of pain.

- It is important to recognize (and adequately address) the presence of other medical comorbidities that impact the patient with mTMD.

DISCLOSURE

The authors have nothing to disclose.

REFERENCES

1. Dahlhamer J, Lucas J, Zelaya C, et al. Prevalence of chronic pain and high-impact chronic pain among adults - United States, 2016. MMWR Morb Mortal Wkly Rep 2018;67(36):1001–6.

2. Fayaz A, Croft P, Langford RM, et al. Prevalence of chronic pain in the UK: a systematic review and meta-analysis of population studies. BMJ Open 2016;6(6): e010364.

3. Slade G, Durham J. Prevalence, impact and costs of treatment for temporomandibular disorders. paper commisioned by the committee on temporomandibular disorders (TMDs): from research discoveries to clinical treatment. In: Temporomandibular disorders: priorities for research and care. Washington, DC: National Academies Press (US); 2020. p. 1–409. ISBN-13: 978-0-309-67048-7 ISBN-10: 0-309-67048-9.

4. Miller VE, Poole C, Golightly Y, et al. Characteristics associated with high-impact pain in people with temporomandibular disorder: a cross-sectional study. J Pain 2019;20(3):288–300.

5. White BA, Williams LA, Leben JR. Health care utilization and cost among health maintenance organization members with temporomandibular disorders. J Orofac Pain 2001;15(2):158–69.

6. Shah JP, Thaker N, Heimur J, et al. Myofascial trigger points then and now: a historical and scientific perspective. PM R 2015;7(7):746–61.

7. Manfredini D, Guarda-Nardini L, Winocur E, et al. Research diagnostic criteria for temporomandibular disorders: a systematic review of axis I epidemiologic findings. Oral Surg Oral Med Oral Pathol Oral Radiol Endod 2011;112(4):453–62.

8. Schiffman E, Ohrbach R, Truelove E, et al. Diagnostic criteria for temporomandibular disorders (DC/TMD) for clinical and research applications: recommendations of the international RDC/TMD consortium network* and orofacial pain special interest Groupdagger. J Oral Facial Pain Headache 2014;28(1):6–27.

9. International classification of orofacial pain, 1st edition (ICOP). Cephalalgia 2020; 40(2):129–221.

10. Ahmad M, Schiffman EL. Temporomandibular joint disorders and orofacial pain. Dent Clin North Am 2016;60(1):105–24.

11. Schiffman E, Ohrbach R. Executive summary of the diagnostic criteria for temporomandibular disorders for clinical and research applications. J Am Dent Assoc 2016;147(6):438–45.

12. Fitzcharles MA, Cohen SP, Clauw DJ, et al. Nociplastic pain: towards an understanding of prevalent pain conditions. Lancet 2021;397(10289):2098–110.

13. Kalladka M, Young A, Khan J. Myofascial pain in temporomandibular disorders: Updates on etiopathogenesis and management. J Bodyw Mov Ther 2021;28: 104–13.

14. Kosek E, Clauw D, Nijs J, et al. Chronic nociplastic pain affecting the musculoskeletal system: clinical criteria and grading system. Pain 2021;162(11):2629–34.

15. Thoma N, Pilecki B, McKay D. Contemporary cognitive behavior therapy: a review of theory, history, and evidence. Psychodyn Psychiatry 2015;43(3):423–61.

16. Noma N, Watanabe Y, Shimada A, et al. Effects of cognitive behavioral therapy on orofacial pain conditions. J Oral Sci 2020;63(1):4–7.

17. Al-Moraissi EA, Farea R, Qasem KA, et al. Effectiveness of occlusal splint therapy in the management of temporomandibular disorders: network meta-analysis of randomized controlled trials. Int J Oral Maxillofac Surg 2020;49(8):1042–56.

18. Al-Moraissi EA, Wolford LM, Ellis E 3rd, et al. The hierarchy of different treatments for arthrogenous temporomandibular disorders: A network meta-analysis of randomized clinical trials. J Craniomaxillofac Surg 2020;48(1):9–23.

19. Serritella E, Galluccio G, Impellizzeri A, et al. Comparison of the effectiveness of three different acupuncture methods for tmd-related pain: a randomized clinical study. Evid Based Complement Alternat Med 2021;2021:1286570.

20. Calixtre LB, Moreira RF, Franchini GH, et al. Manual therapy for the management of pain and limited range of motion in subjects with signs and symptoms of temporomandibular disorder: a systematic review of randomised controlled trials. J Oral Rehabil 2015;42(11):847–61.

21. Bialosky JE, Bishop MD, Price DD, et al. The mechanisms of manual therapy in the treatment of musculoskeletal pain: a comprehensive model. Man Ther 2009;14(5):531–8.

22. Sobral APT, Godoy CLH, Fernandes KPS, et al. Photomodulation in the treatment of chronic pain in patients with temporomandibular disorder: protocol for cost-effectiveness analysis. BMJ Open 2018;8(5):e018326.

23. Xu GZ, Jia J, Jin L, et al. Low-level laser therapy for temporomandibular disorders: a systematic review with meta-analysis. Pain Res Manag 2018;2018: 4230583.

24. Gerwin RD. Myofascial trigger point pain syndromes. Semin Neurol 2016;36(5): 469–73.

25. Al-Moraissi EA, Alradom J, Aladashi O, et al. Needling therapies in the management of myofascial pain of the masticatory muscles: A network meta-analysis of randomised clinical trials. J Oral Rehabil 2020;47(7):910–22.

26. Dunning J, Butts R, Mourad F, et al. Dry needling: a literature review with implications for clinical practice guidelines. Phys Ther Rev 2014;19(4):252–65.

27. Fernandes G, Goncalves DAG, Conti P. Musculoskeletal disorders. Dent Clin North Am 2018;62(4):553–64.

28. Vincent MB, Luna RA, Scandiuzzi D, et al. Greater occipital nerve blockade in cervicogenic headache. Arq Neuropsiquiatr 1998;56(4):720–5.

29. Saadah HA, Taylor FB. Sustained headache syndrome associated with tender occipital nerve zones. Headache 1987;27(4):201–5.

30. Ananthan S, Kanti V, Zagury JG, et al. The effect of the twin block compared with trigger point injections in patients with masticatory myofascial pain: a pilot study. Oral Surg Oral Med Oral Pathol Oral Radiol 2020;129(3):222–8.

31. Kanti V, Ananthan S, Subramanian G, et al. Efficacy of the twin block, a peripheral nerve block for the management of chronic masticatory myofascial pain: A case series. Quintessence Int 2017;725–9.

32. Quek S, Young A, Subramanian G. The twin block: a simple technique to block both the masseteric and the anterior deep temporal nerves with one anesthetic injection. Oral Surg Oral Med Oral Pathol Oral Radiol 2014;118(3):e65–7.

33. Quek SYP, Gomes-Zagury J, Subramanian G. Twin block in myogenous orofacial pain: applied anatomy, technique update, and safety. Anesth Prog 2020;67(2): 103–6.

34. Subramanian GaQ, SYP. Temporo-masseteric nerve block impairs efferent conduction to temporalis and masseter. 51st AADOCR/CADR Annual Meeting & Exhibition; 2022.

35. Mujakperuo HR, Watson M, Morrison R, et al. Pharmacological interventions for pain in patients with temporomandibular disorders. Cochrane Database Syst Rev 2010;10:CD004715.

36. Knotkova H, Hamani C, Sivanesan E, et al. Neuromodulation for chronic pain. Lancet 2021;397(10289):2111–24.

37. Korwisi B, Garrido Suarez BB, Goswami S, et al. Reliability and clinical utility of the chronic pain classification in the 11th Revision of the International Classification of Diseases from a global perspective: results from India, Cuba, and New Zealand. Pain 2022;163(3):e453–62.

38. Fernandes AC, Duarte Moura DM, Da Silva LGD, et al. Acupuncture in Temporo-mandibular Disorder Myofascial Pain Treatment: A Systematic Review. J Oral Facial Pain Headache 2017;31(3):225–32.

39. Ozden MCP, Atalay B Dds MP, Ozden Av Dds P, et al. Efficacy of dry needling in patients with myofascial temporomandibular disorders related to the masseter muscle. Cranio 2020;38(5):305–11.

40. de Melo LA, Bezerra de Medeiros AK, Campos M, et al. Manual therapy in the treatment of myofascial pain related to temporomandibular disorders: a system-atic review. J Oral Facial Pain Headache 2020;34(2):141–8.

41. Ahmad SA, Hasan S, Saeed S, et al. Low-level laser therapy in temporomandib-ular joint disorders: a systematic review. J Med Life 2021;14(2):148–64.

42. Kuc J, Szarejko KD, Golebiewska M. Evaluation of soft tissue mobilization in pa-tients with temporomandibular disorder-myofascial pain with referral. Int J Environ Res Public Health 2020;17(24):9576.

43. Serritella E, Scialanca G, Di Giacomo P, et al. Local vibratory stimulation for temporomandibular disorder myofascial pain treatment: a randomised, double-blind, placebo-controlled preliminary study. Pain Res Manag 2020;2020: 6705307.

44. Roldan-Barraza C, Janko S, Villanueva J, et al. A systematic review and meta-analysis of usual treatment versus psychosocial interventions in the treatment of myofascial temporomandibular disorder pain. J Oral Facial Pain Headache 2014;28(3):205–22.

45. Giannakopoulos NN, Rauer AK, Hellmann D, et al. Comparison of device-supported sensorimotor training and splint intervention for myofascial temporo-mandibular disorder pain patients. J Oral Rehabil 2018;45(9):669–76.

46. van Grootel RJ, Buchner R, Wismeijer D, et al. Towards an optimal therapy strat-egy for myogenous TMD, physiotherapy compared with occlusal splint therapy in an RCT with therapy-and-patient-specific treatment durations. BMC Musculoske-let Disord 2017;18(1):76.

47. Bair E, Brownstein NC, Ohrbach R, et al. Study protocol, sample characteristics, and loss to follow-up: the OPPERA prospective cohort study. J Pain 2013;14(12 Suppl):T2–19.

48. Slade GD, Fillingim RB, Sanders AE, et al. Summary of findings from the OPPERA prospective cohort study of incidence of first-onset temporomandibular disorder: implications and future directions. J Pain 2013;14(12 Suppl):T116–24.

49. National Academies of Sciences E, Medicine. Temporomandibular disorders: pri-orities for research and care. Washington, DC: The National Academies Press; 2020.

50. Glette M, Stiles TC, Borchgrevink PC, et al. The natural course of chronic pain in a general population: stability and change in an eight-wave longitudinal study over four years (the HUNT Pain Study). J Pain 2020;21(5–6):689–99.

51. Ibrahim T, Tleyjeh IM, Gabbar O. Surgical versus non-surgical treatment of chronic low back pain: a meta-analysis of randomised trials. Int Orthop 2008; 32(1):107–13.

52. Initiative NH. Quantitative Evaluation of Myofascial Tissues: Potential Impact for Musculoskeletal Pain Research. Paper presented at: NIH HEAL Inititiative Work-shop on Myofascial Pain2020. September 16, 2020 - 08:45 a.m. ET to September 17, 2020 3:30 p.m. ET Zoom and NIH Videocast. Available at: https://www.nccih. nih.gov/news/events/nih-heal-initiative-workshop-on-myofascial-pain.

53. Volkow N, Benveniste H, McLellan AT. Use and misuse of opioids in chronic pain. Annu Rev Med 2018;69:451–65.

54. Koutris M, Lobbezoo F, Sumer NC, et al. Is myofascial pain in temporomandibular disorder patients a manifestation of delayed-onset muscle soreness? Clin J Pain 2013;29(8):712–6.
55. Wilke J, Behringer M. Is "delayed onset muscle soreness" a false friend? the potential implication of the fascial connective tissue in post-exercise discomfort. Int J Mol Sci 2021;22(17):9482.
56. Stecco A, Gesi M, Stecco C, et al. Fascial components of the myofascial pain syndrome. Curr Pain Headache Rep 2013;17(8):352.
57. Ettlin DA, Napimoga MH, Meira ECM, et al. Orofacial musculoskeletal pain: An evidence-based bio-psycho-social matrix model. Neurosci Biobehav Rev 2021; 128:12–20.
58. Manfredini D, Lobbezoo F. Relationship between bruxism and temporomandibular disorders: a systematic review of literature from 1998 to 2008. Oral Surg Oral Med Oral Pathol Oral Radiol Endod 2010;109(6):e26–50.
59. Bucci R, Lobbezoo F, Michelotti A, et al. Two repetitive bouts of intense eccentric-concentric jaw exercises reduce experimental muscle pain in healthy subjects. J Oral Rehabil 2018;45(8):575–80.
60. Fillingim RB, Slade GD, Greenspan JD, et al. Long-term changes in biopsychosocial characteristics related to temporomandibular disorder: findings from the OPPERA study. Pain 2018;159(11):2403–13.
61. Louca Jounger S, Christidis N, Svensson P, et al. Increased levels of intramuscular cytokines in patients with jaw muscle pain. J Headache Pain 2017;18(1):30.
62. Fricton J. Myofascial pain: mechanisms to management. Oral Maxillofacial Surg Clin N Am 2016;28(3):289–311.
63. Shrivastava M, Battaglino R, Ye L. A comprehensive review on biomarkers associated with painful temporomandibular disorders. Int J Oral Sci 2021;13(1):23.
64. Sessle BJ. Chronic orofacial pain: models, mechanisms, and genetic and related environmental influences. Int J Mol Sci 2021;22(13):7112.
65. Slade GD, Ohrbach R, Greenspan JD, et al. Painful temporomandibular disorder: decade of discovery from OPPERA studies. J Dent Res 2016;95(10):1084–92.
66. Ernberg M, Jasim H, Wahlen K, et al. Altered plasma proteins in myogenous temporomandibular disorders. J Clin Med 2022;11(10):2777.
67. Duarte FCK, West DWD, Linde LD, et al. Re-examining myofascial pain syndrome: toward biomarker development and mechanism-based diagnostic criteria. Curr Rheumatol Rep 2021;23(8):69.
68. Madariaga VI, Jasim H, Ghafouri B, et al. Myogenous temporomandibular disorders and salivary markers of oxidative stress-A cross-sectional study. J Oral Rehabil 2021;48(1):1–9.
69. Jasim H, Ghafouri B, Gerdle B, et al. Altered levels of salivary and plasma pain related markers in temporomandibular disorders. J Headache Pain 2020; 21(1):105.
70. Pillen S, Boon A, Van Alfen N. Muscle ultrasound. Handb Clin Neurol 2016;136: 843–53.
71. Barkhordarian A, Demerjian G, Chiappelli F. Translational research of temporomandibular joint pathology: a preliminary biomarker and fMRI study. J Transl Med 2020;18(1):22.
72. Moayedi M, Hodaie M. Trigeminal nerve and white matter brain abnormalities in chronic orofacial pain disorders. Pain Rep 2019;4(4):e755.
73. Nastro E, Bonanno L, Catalfamo L, et al. Diffusion tensor imaging reveals morphological alterations of the lateral pterygoid muscle in patients with mandibular asymmetry. Dentomaxillofac Radiol 2018;47(1):20170129.

74. Suenaga S, Nagayama K, Nagasawa T, et al. The usefulness of diagnostic imaging for the assessment of pain symptoms in temporomandibular disorders. Jpn Dent Sci Rev 2016;52(4):93–106.

75. Karlsson L, Gerdle B, Ghafouri B, et al. Intramuscular pain modulatory substances before and after exercise in women with chronic neck pain. Eur J Pain 2015;19(8):1075–85.

76. Louca S, Christidis N, Ghafouri B, et al. Serotonin, glutamate and glycerol are released after the injection of hypertonic saline into human masseter muscles - a microdialysis study. J Headache Pain 2014;15:89.

77. Dawson A, Ghafouri B, Gerdle B, et al. Effects of experimental tooth clenching on pain and intramuscular release of 5-HT and glutamate in patients with myofascial TMD. Clin J Pain 2015;31(8):740–9.

78. Dawson A, Ghafouri B, Gerdle B, et al. Pain and intramuscular release of algesic substances in the masseter muscle after experimental tooth-clenching exercises in healthy subjects. J Orofac Pain 2013;27(4):350–60.

79. Bron C, Dommerholt JD. Etiology of myofascial trigger points. Curr Pain Headache Rep 2012;16(5):439–44.

80. Cao QW, Peng BG, Wang L, et al. Expert consensus on the diagnosis and treatment of myofascial pain syndrome. World J Clin Cases 2021;9(9):2077–89.

81. Sikdar S, Shah JP, Gebreab T, et al. Novel applications of ultrasound technology to visualize and characterize myofascial trigger points and surrounding soft tissue. Arch Phys Med Rehabil 2009;90(11):1829–38.

82. Hotta N, Kubo A, Mizumura K. Chondroitin sulfate attenuates acid-induced augmentation of the mechanical response in rat thin-fiber muscle afferents in vitro. J Appl Physiol (1985) 2019;126(4):1160–70.

Temporomandibular Disorders: Surgical Implications and Management

Peter Henein, DMD*, Vincent B. Ziccardi, DDS, MD

KEYWORDS

- Temporomandibular disorder • Arthrocentesis • Arthroscopy
- Total joint replacement • Temporomandibular joint

KEY POINTS

- Temporomandibular disorders have multiple management options, and the goal is to eliminate pain and restore function.
- When temporomandibular disorders fail, conservative therapy, noninvasive surgery, and open joint surgery should be explored.
- Arthrocentesis and arthroscopy can achieve predictable results for Wilkes Class II and III patients.
- Total joint replacement is reserved for Wilkes Class IV and V patients with limited function and can predictably restore a functional maximal incisal opening.

INTRODUCTION

Temporomandibular disorders (TMDs) are among the most common pain disorders in the United States. General dentists are in the forefront of screening, diagnosing, and referring these patients to specialists who can offer treatment modalities to eliminate pain and facilitate a return to normal function. The spectrum of TMDs is broad and treatments exist which vary greatly in their invasiveness. Therefore, appropriate diagnosis is critical before initiating surgical treatment. TMDs that are extra-articular in origin are generally treated nonsurgically. Management modalities include physical therapy, pharmacotherapy, and occlusal appliance therapy. Internal derangements can also be treated nonsurgically, and if nonresponsive, surgical management can be considered. Nonsurgical management of internal derangements includes pharmacotherapy, physical therapy, occlusal splint therapy, and lifestyle adaptations.

Intra-articular diseases such as rheumatoid arthritis, osteoarthritis, recurrent dislocation, ankylosis, and other intracapsular pathologies may require surgical

Department of Oral and Maxillofacial Surgery, Rutgers School of Dental Medicine, 110 Bergen Street, Room B854, Newark, NJ 07103-2400, USA
* Corresponding author.
E-mail address: ph219@sdm.rutgers.edu

Dent Clin N Am 67 (2023) 349–365
https://doi.org/10.1016/j.cden.2022.12.002
0011-8532/23/© 2022 Elsevier Inc. All rights reserved.

intervention for adequate management.[1] The surgical procedures to be discussed in this article range from minimally invasive procedures such as arthrocentesis and arthroscopy to open joint surgery including disc plication and repositioning and osseous surgery such as condylotomy and eminoplasty. When all other nonsurgical and surgical modalities have failed, in most treatment algorithms, a prosthetic total joint replacement (TJR) is then resorted to. The goal of this article is to review the various surgical modalities, so that the general dentist, oral and maxillofacial surgeon, orofacial pain specialist, and other health care providers can work together to provide patient-centered care and optimal outcomes.

Patient Evaluation

Patient evaluation begins with a comprehensive review of medical history, medications, and review of systems. The provider should pay close attention to pertinent positive responses that are concerning for underlying systemic issues that may contribute to TMD. The next step is a thorough head and neck examination. Physical examination involves a full review of the joint, masticatory muscle system, and range of functional movements including any parafunctional habits. The patient should be examined for any hypertrophy or abnormalities of the bones or muscles as well as any facial asymmetry, which may alert the clinician of a history of trauma or other pathological condition. The muscles should be palpated to evaluate for tenderness and trigger points. The temporomandibular joint (TMJ) is palpated for tenderness at rest. The patient should be instructed to open and close their mouth while the dentist rests their hands on the joints, carefully feeling for clicking or crepitus of the joint, paying close attention to when the clicking occurs. The midline of the mandible should be examined during opening and closing to check for any deviation or deflection. Next, the range of motion should be examined and recorded. Normal mandibular opening is greater than 40 mm, with lateral and protrusive movements measuring approximately 8 to 10 mm.[2] If a patient is noted to have limited movement in any direction, the clinician should provide gentle pressure to encourage further movement. This will help provide information as to whether the limitation is from an intracapsular structural derangement or from muscular pain. Finally, the dentition should be evaluated for wear facets and signs of bruxism or other parafunctional habits. Protrusive and lateral contacts should be examined to determine whether interferences are present. Occlusal contacts in centric and functional movements are evaluated using articulating article. Otoscopic examination is performed to ascertain any pathology or perforations of the tympanic membrane, which may be source of referred pain. Radiographic evaluation provides important information about the joint and helps guide the clinician in classification and potential treatment options (**Fig. 1**). Plain films and panoramic radiographs are appropriate screening tools for limited TMJ evaluation, whereas computer tomography is the gold standard for evaluating bony anatomy.

Classification of Temporomandibular Joint Disorders

All of the above tools used together will guide the clinician on diagnosis and classification of TMDs. Myofascial pain disorder (MFPD) is the most common diagnosis associated with muscular pain, tenderness in masticatory muscles during palpation, and sometimes decreased range of motion.[3] Headaches may also be associated. Of note, MFPD is usually exacerbated by stress and excessive function. Radiographic evaluation is generally unremarkable. Internal derangements involve abnormal disk function. Usually, the articular disk follows the mandibular condyle during function and will glide down the articular eminence anteriorly with the condylar head. The intermediate zone remains in contact with the superior aspect of the condylar head during

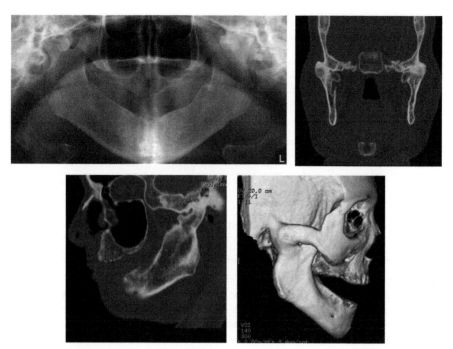

Fig. 1. Radiographic images showing bilateral bony ankylosis of the TMJ. Notice how the condylar bone is fused to the fossa.

rest and during maximal opening. Anterior disk displacement with reduction means that the disk is anteromedially displaced at rest and then shifts into normal position between the condylar head and glenoid fossa during opening (reduction). Clicking will generally be heard and palpated both during displacement and reduction. Computed tomography (CT) evaluation of these patients is generally unremarkable, whereas MRI will clearly show the disk anteriorly displaced during the closed position. Anterior displacement without reduction is a more advanced stage of internal derangement, where the disk is displaced anteromedially at rest, but does not reduce with maximal opening. No clicking is heard, as the disk does not reduce. On examination, these patients will have mandibular deviation to the affected side, with decreased opening and decreased lateral excursion to the contralateral side. MRI will reveal disk displacement in both the closed and open position. The Wilkes classification provides five stages of internal derangement of the TMJ and is useful in identifying and standardizing the extent of disease. **Table 1** shows the Wilkes Classification by clinical and radiographic changes.

Degenerative joint disease (DJD) results in bony abnormalities including flattening of the condylar head and the presence of osteophytes. Osteophytes are bony spurs that develop in the joint space as a host adaptive response during late stages of TMD.[4] The process of DJD is the same compared with other joints and is described as a disease of "wear and tear." Excessive stress on joints leads to hypoxia and the production of oxygen-free radicals, which are damaging to the cells of the joint. The release of inflammatory cytokines such as prostaglandins and leukotrienes also contribute to degeneration of the joint. Patients with DJD fall under Wilkes stages IV and V, as they have remodeling of the bones of the joint. These patients may present with pain and crepitus of the joint and limited movement. Crepitus may be felt as vibration during opening or auscultated with a stethoscope as the sound of Velcro opening.

Table 1		
Wilkes staging classification for internal derangement of the temporomandibular joint		
Stage	**Clinical**	**Radiographic**
Stage I	+/− painless clicking, no pain, no limited function	No osseous changes, slight anterior disk displacement
Stage II	Mild occasional pain, clicking	No osseous changes, slight anterior disk displacement and early signs of deformity of disk
Stage III	Frequent pain, limited function, locking, painful chewing	Normal osseous contours, anterior disk displacement, thickening of the posterior disk
Stage IV	Chronic pain, headaches, limited range of motion	Degenerative osseous changes, anterior disk displacement, thickening of posterior disk
Stage V	Crepitus, limited opening, difficulty with eating	Gross disk deformity including perforation, severe degenerative osseous changes, and osteophytes

Rheumatoid arthritis patients present with similar findings to DJD, but the etiology is different. Systemic signs of inflammation are present and multiple joints may be affected. Rheumatoid arthritis is generally bilateral, whereas DJD is generally unilateral. Radiographic examination may reveal degeneration of the bones of the joint, and the destruction can generally be more severe and involve erosion of the condylar head. These patients may progress to requiring TJR with prosthetic joints in advanced cases.

Hypermobility of the joint will allow the condylar head to advance beyond the articular eminence and become locked beyond the eminence. This is called dislocation, which may occur during yawning or eating. Reduction of the dislocation is completed with downward and posterior pressure on the posterior teeth and may be aided with local anesthesia of masticatory muscles and/or IV sedation. Patient who have recurrent dislocation can be treated with eminoplasty, a procedure to flatten out the articular eminence. This essentially allows patients to dislocate and relocate freely. This is in contrast to those patients whose condyle dislocates beyond the anterior aspect of the articular eminence, but self-reduces in a process called subluxation.

Ankylosis of the TMJ (**Fig.1**) involves fusion of the condyle to the temporal bones. Patients with TMJ ankylosis will present with severely limited mobility. This fusion may be fibrous, bony, or a combination of both. These patients may have had a history of trauma, specifically condylar fractures which were not reduced, resulting in bleeding in the joint with subsequent lack of movement, creating fibrous and bony adhesions. For this reason, early mobility is prioritized in treatment of condylar fractures to prevent adhesions. Infection of the joint, including spread from middle ear infections, can also lead to hypomobility and ankylosis, especially in children, if untreated. Growth disturbances will be noted, causing deviation toward the affected side from unrestricted growth of the normal contralateral joint. Neoplasms of the TMJ are rare, but when they do occur, they present with TMD symptoms such as pain and restricted movement in the joint. CT will generally show abnormality of the affected joint.

Surgical Procedures for Temporomandibular Joint Disorders

Arthrocentesis

TMJ arthrocentesis is a minimally invasive surgical treatment option that can be offered to patients with internal derangement of the joint and other inflammatory arthropathies which are unresponsive to nonsurgical management. Major indications for arthrocentesis are acute or chronic pain with limited range of motion due to disk displacement (with or without reduction). Nitzan and colleagues reported long-term success on 39 out of 40 patients who presented with acute closed lock and were treated with arthrocentesis.[5] After 16.6 months, patients had significant improvement in pain and dysfunction, and no patients had recurrence of their closed lock.[5] This procedure generally has a low morbidity, short surgical time, and patients go home the same day. Some surgeons perform this procedure in the office with intra venous (IV) sedation, whereas others prefer the operating room, with general anesthesia to allow for jaw manipulation while the muscles are fully relaxed. For these reasons, arthrocentesis is a reasonable first-line therapy to a patient with more extensive DJD, before considering open joint procedures. Some patients will experience a decrease in pain and enough function to return to activities of daily life without more invasive surgery or the procedure can be repeated at a later date for symptomatic relief. Contraindications to arthrocentesis are patients with limited mobility without pain due to fibrous or bony ankylosis.

The procedure involves lavage of the upper joint space and the use of hydraulic pressure and manipulation to release jaw adhesions. The superior joint space is identified at a point 10 mm anterior and 2 mm inferior to the anterior portion of the external auditory meatus on a line drawn from the lateral canthus to the tragus of the ear (**Figs. 2** and **3**). An inflow needle is placed in the superior joint space at this point and fluid is injected. Although the joint is insufflated, an outflow needle is then placed in the prominence of the articular eminence, and thorough lavage of the joint is completed by flushing 100 to 200 mL of lactated Ringer solution through the joint. Studies by Kanayema and Gulen[6,7] evaluated 17 joints that had undergone arthrocentesis and noted that with 200 mL of irrigant, the levels of bradykinin and interleukin-6 was significantly decreased, and that with 300 to 400 mL, the cytokines were no longer detectable in the joint fluid. The jaw should be manipulated during the procedure, allowing release of adhesions. At the conclusion of the procedure, various medicaments can be injected into the joint including steroids, opioids, synthetic hyaluronic acid, and platelet-rich plasma.

The rationale behind the effectiveness arthrocentesis is not well understood, but multiple hypotheses exist. The procedure does not mechanically alter any of the causes of internal derangement, but does alleviate the symptoms.[8] When disk displacement occurs, negative pressure occurs within the joint, similar to a suction cup. Insufflating the joint eliminates this suction cup effect. Irrigation and lavage of the joint may release some minor adhesions present between the disk and the fossa. Chemical mediators of inflammation are also flushed away during the procedure, and injection of steroids helps break the cycle.[9] Some patients have been reported to have a closed lock (anterior disk displacement without reduction) converted into disk displacement *with* reduction, which leads to improved function and a decrease in pain.[10] Postoperative passive motion is critical to prevent the reformation of any adhesions, stimulate production of synovial fluid, and clear any blood in the joint from the procedure. Patients should continue to wear occlusal appliances, participate in physical therapy, and use medications as appropriate including NSAIDS and/or muscle relaxants as prescribed.

Arthroscopy

Arthroscopy is the next-level surgical procedure which has the benefits of arthrocentesis with visualization and options for advanced procedures using an additional port.[11] The most common arthroscopic procedure is lysis and lavage, which is essentially the

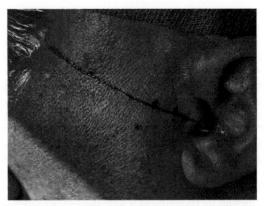

Fig. 2. Cantho-tragal line with markings for arthrocentesis/arthroscopy. The dots mark the locations where the inflow and outflow portals will be placed.

same as completing an arthrocentesis, but with direct visualization of the joint.[12,13] Arthroscopy can also be an operative procedure through which biopsy, adhesion removal, and disc repositioning can be performed.[9] **Fig. 4** shows the armamentarium for an arthroscopy, including the arthroscope and trocar. The same markings as an arthrocentesis are used for joint access (see **Fig. 9**). After injecting local anesthesia into the joint, a small incision is made in the skin overlying the superior joint space, a trocar is inserted into the joint, and then the camera is placed. A second outflow port is established to flush the joint during examination, enhancing visualization. At this point, the medial capsule and fibers of the lateral pterygoid muscle will be visualized (**Fig. 5**). The camera can then be moved to visualize all aspects of the joint, especially the disk and retrodiscal tissue. Abnormal findings include increased vascularity, hyperemic tissue, and compressed retrodiscal tissue.[13] Adhesions and fibrillations can also be visualized throughout the examination and released with blunt trocar sweep. **Fig. 6** demonstrates fibrillations and minor erythema of the joint space. **Fig. 7** exhibits calcified adhesions of the joint with extensive fibrillations. After examination, the scope is advanced to the most anterior and lateral portion of the joint. The skin will be transilluminated and the cannula is inserted in this position. The operator

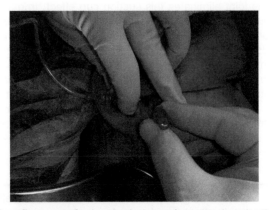

Fig. 3. Inflow and outflow ports for lavage during arthrocentesis. Irrigation will be flushed through the joint and should freely flow out of the outflow port.

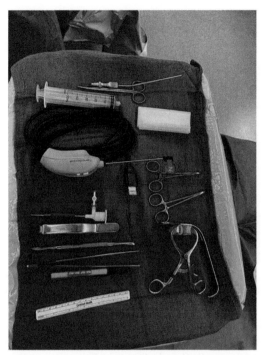

Fig. 4. Armamentarium for arthroscopy including the arthroscope, marking pen, ruler, syringe for irrigation, and instruments for dissection.

can observe the lysis and lavage (**Fig. 8**), and if desired, instruments can be introduced through an additional puncture site. Various knives, shavers, and lasers can be used to break down adhesions under direct visualization.[11] Biopsy of tissue can be taken if there is any concern for pathology. Further, discopexy can be completed with a

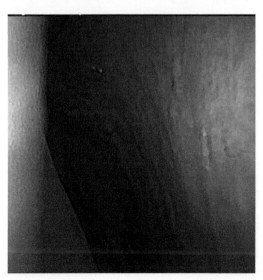

Fig. 5. Arthroscopic view of the joint. This joint is clear with no fibrillations or erythema.

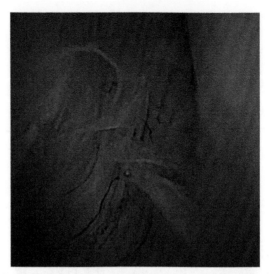

Fig. 6. Arthroscopic view of the joint with fibrillations and erythema. The white web-like adhesions are fibrillations which should be broken up during the procedure if possible.

goal to reposition the disk posteriorly in its proper anatomic position in cases of anterior disc displacement.[12] This is accomplished by performing an anterior release where the lateral pterygoid attaches to the disk. This releases the anteromedial pull and allows the disk to be repositioned posteriorly. The disk reduction is held in place using a suture or tack. Alternatively, a laser can be used to contract the tissues posteriorly, thereby pulling the disk posteriorly. Complications are similar to those of arthrocentesis including damage to the fifth and seventh cranial nerves, which resolves spontaneously in almost all cases. Carter demonstrated that the incidence of

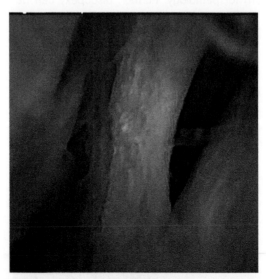

Fig. 7. Calcified adhesions of joint and fibrillations. These adhesions are consistent with limited mouth opening and pain during function.

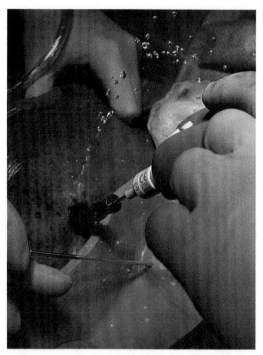

Fig. 8. Lavage irrigation during arthroscopy. Notice how freely the water is flowing out as it freely passes through the joint space.

vascular damage was about 2% in these procedures, and hemorrhage can be controlled with electrocautery or pressure in most cases.[14] On completion of arthroscopy, various substances can be injected into the superior joint space, similar to arthrocentesis.

Condylotomy
Condylotomy is a surgical procedure that does not involve opening the joint.[15] This extracapsular procedure was popularized by Hall, who described this procedure in an article involving 190 patients and 305 joints with success rates of 70% to 80%.[16] The procedure involves an intraoral vertical osteotomy in the ramus, posterior to the lingula. This allows the proximal segment, which contains the condyle, to sag inferiorly. When the condyle sags inferiorly (about 1.5 to 3 mm), the compression on the disk and retrodiscal tissues is decreased to potentially allow disc repositioning. Pain is reduced because the disk has space to reduce into the proper position. No bony fixation is used, but patients are placed in maxillomandibular fixation for one to two weeks, followed by four to six weeks of elastics with joint mobility and training exercises. The advantage of this procedure is that it is extracapsular, eliminating the risks of open joint surgery and the subsequent scarring in the joint space and potential for facial nerve injury.

Arthroplasty
Arthroplasty is reserved for patients with TMJ pain and dysfunction that has failed to improve after conservative and arthroscopic treatment.[10] The goal is to decrease pain and increase functional movements. Various techniques include disc repositioning, disc repair, discectomy with or without grafting, and gap arthroplasty. The surgical

approaches to the joint include an endaural incision or preauricular incision.[17] The preauricular incision is most commonly used and involves a 3 cm long vertical incision directly anterior to the tragus of the ear in a natural skin crease. The skin and subcutaneous tissues are sharply dissected down to the temporoparietal fascia. The superficial temporal artery and vein may be ligated at this point if they are encountered. The superficial and deep layer of the deep temporal fascia is separated by temporal extension of the buccal fat pad. Superior to the zygomatic arch, the superficial layer of the deep temporal fascia is sharply dissected at a 45° angle (parallel to the course of the facial nerve) approximately 2 cm above the zygomatic arch. Blunt dissection below this layer is completed until the zygomatic arch is encountered. Sharp dissection is completed to release the periosteum off the zygomatic arch, which will then allow the articular eminence to be visualized with retraction of tissue in a subperiosteal plane. The superior joint capsule is then visualized. The mandible can be manipulated at this time to verify the lateral pole of the condyle. The joint can then be entered by sharply dissecting through the joint capsule after insufflating the joint with fluid, exposing the superior joint space. To enter the inferior joint space, an inferior incision is made on the neck of the condyle and the disk will be visualized. Disc integrity and position should be identified before manipulation. If the disk is intact and has a normal appearance, chances are higher that disc repositioning procedures will succeed. Disc imbrication refers to removing a small wedge of posterior tissue to allow the disk to be repositioned posteriorly, if it is displaced anteriorly. The wedge of tissue is removed and then the disk is sutured back together. Plication is defined as pulling the disc posteriorly and folding on itself to suture in place and can be performed with potentially less morbidity. Disc repair can be completed if any perforations through the disk are noted. Perforations most commonly occur at the junction of the posterior disk and retrodiscal tissues.[18] This involves freeing the disk superiorly and inferiorly first with direct repair of small perforations primarily with sutures. Discectomy is reserved for deformed disks that are beyond repair. Only the central portion of the disk and some of the posterior band is usually removed, leaving behind the most vascular retrodiscal tissues and anterior attachment. After the disk has been removed, irregular bony contours can be remodeled using hand and rotary instruments. Takaku and Toyoda's study followed 39 patients who had discectomy and were followed for 20 years; 37 patients had no more pain and achieved 35 mm of mouth opening.[19] Eriksson and Westesson's study also followed 15 discectomy patients for 29 years and had similar results, with only one patient who achieved less than 39 mm of opening.[20] The bones undergo significant remodeling after this procedure, and patients usually have flattening of the fossa and condyle radiographically, but this is not significant if associated without pain or dysfunction. Patients may experience temporary occlusal changes due to change in vertical dimension which usually resolves over time. Discectomy can also include replacement tissues to be placed in between the condyle and fossa to prevent joint adhesion. The materials used for disc replacement are temporalis muscle/fascia, auricular cartilage, dermis, and abdominal fat.

Gap arthroplasty is another procedure that can be used to treat TMJ ankylosis. The surgery involves creating a gap at the level of the joint space. The TMJ is exposed and identified (**Fig. 9**). The bony ankylosed segment is excised, creating a joint space followed by removal of the coronoid process (**Fig. 10**). **Fig. 11** shows a fat graft that is placed in the gap to prevent recurrence of the ankylosis and osteophyte formation. The remaining gap between the glenoid fossa and mandible should be at least 15 mm. This has been shown to allow at least 30 mm of incisal opening.[21] A study by Roychoudhury and colleagues[22] demonstrated that in 50 patients treated by gap arthroplasty, the mean maximal incisal opening after 36 months was 30.62 mm.

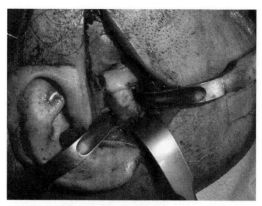

Fig. 9. Through a pre-auricular incision, the joint is accessed and a true bony ankylosis is seen.

Eminoplasty, used for the treatment of hypermobility, is another important adjunct in the surgical correction of internal derangements and TMJ pathology.[23] The procedure can be completed arthroscopically with comparable success rates, but most surgeons prefer the open technique for better visualization.[24] TMJ dislocation occurs when the condyle translates anteriorly beyond the articular eminence and cannot be self-reduced. Patients who have frequent dislocation may be treated with eminoplasty to allow the joint to freely translate. Imaging should be reviewed before the procedure to ensure that bony removal of the eminence will not result in intracranial exposure of the temporal lobe. A fissure bur can be used to score the osteotomy to the level of the zygomatic process. The osteotomy is completed with a sharp osteotomy angled slightly inferiorly. A reciprocating rasp is then used to flatten and smooth the remaining bone. **Fig. 12** shows an intraoperative photograph of a zygomatic arch after eminoplasty has been completed. Some surgeons advocate for two weeks of intermaxillary fixation to encourage scarring and hypomobility of the joint in treating hypermobility. Undt reviewed seven articles that studied recurrent TMJ dislocation following eminoplasty and showed recurrence rates ranging from 0% to 27%.[25] A study by Williamson and McNamara showed that eminoplasty can be used to treat patients with closed

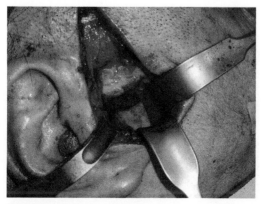

Fig. 10. After the arthroplasty, the bony fusion has been removed and a gap is created between the condylar head and the fossa.

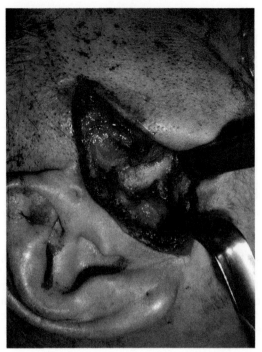

Fig. 11. Fat graft after arthroplasty. The fat is placed in the joint space and will help prevent further bone formation.

lock: maximal incisal opening improved by an average of 12 mm and symptoms improved in 85% of patients. It is the author's practice to include eminoplasty using reciprocating rasp with all arthroplasty procedures to facilitate oral opening and function.

Temporomandibular Joint Replacement

TJR is a complex surgery where the entire joint and bony components are removed and replaced with prosthetic components. Indications for TJR include bony

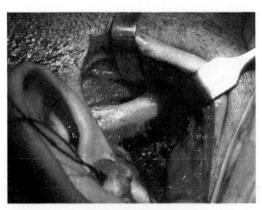

Fig. 12. The articular eminence is seen here after arthroplasty. The eminence is no longer prominent, and the joint can freely translate anteriorly and posteriorly.

ankylosis,[26] pathology involving the joint, idiopathic condylar resorption, severe DJD, avascular necrosis, loss of vertical ramus height with occlusal changes as a result of trauma or bony resorption, and incomplete joint formation due to craniofacial syndromes (hemifacial macrosomia, Treacher Collins, and so forth). In the case of ankylosis, severely limited motion should be present before surgery. Patients can reasonably expect up to 30 mm of opening,[26,27] and this should be achieved immediately intraoperatively, once the prosthesis is in place. Differing opinions exist on TMJ replacement options for the pediatric patient. Some surgeons advocate the use of alloplastic materials to reconstruct the joint to accommodate for the continual growth of the patient; however, subsequent surgical replacement may be required due to growth. Costochondral grafts are primarily used due to the similar dimensions and ability to withstand the forces of mandibular movement and allow for continued condylar growth.[28] The disadvantages include possibility for resorption, ankylosis, and unpredictable growth, and donor-site morbidity. A long-term study by Perrott and colleagues included seven growing patients treated with costochondral TMJ replacement: three of them developed lateral contour overgrowth in the ipsilateral side and none of them developed excessive linear overgrowth resulting in malocclusion.[28]

In the adult patient, alloplastic materials are preferred for joint replacement. Advantages over autogenous grafts include the lack of donor-site morbidity, decreased surgical time, immediate function, and the ability to correct or change occlusion. Stock joints have materials that must be shaped and fitted intraoperatively, whereas custom joints are planned ahead of time and custom milled. The main advantage of stock joints is that they are available immediately and have a significantly lower cost. That being said, more surgeons are moving toward custom joint prosthesis to improve predictability of achieving optimal surgical outcomes.[29] The workflow for planning these surgeries is beyond the scope of this article; however, it is important to note that the workflows exist as one-stage versus two-stage surgeries. In patients where preoperative occlusion is accurate, reproducible, and will not change, surgery can be done in one stage. However, in patients where pathology with malocclusion or other significant mandibular deformity is present, there may be advantages to a two-staged surgery. With the osteotomy and joint removed in the first procedure, the patient can then be placed into maxillomandibular fixation, and a CT scan taken, with the joint then virtually planned. Most centers, however, perform TJR as single-stage procedure, using virtual surgical planning.

In either case, the surgical procedure is the same. Surgery necessitates a preauricular or endaural incision to access the joint and a submandibular incision below the angle of the mandible to access the inferior ramus. With the condyle then exposed, the medial tissues are protected to avoid damage to the internal maxillary artery. A fissure bur or reciprocating saw is used to make a horizontal cut in the condylar neck. Osteotomy is completed with a T-bar osteotomy and the condyle is removed. The glenoid fossa is then prepared and recontoured to accept the prosthetic fossa component. The fossa component is then fitted to place and secured with multiple screws into the zygoma (**Fig. 13**). The patient is then placed into maxillomandibular fixation, and the ramus/condyle unit is fixated to its position into the mandible (**Fig. 14**). The maxillomandibular fixation is then released, and function is assessed intraoperatively before closing the wounds. **Fig. 15** shows postoperative imaging for a patient who underwent bilateral TJR.

Postoperative care is important for these patients. Wound care, elastic therapy, and liquid diet are important for the first 2 to 3 weeks. Physical therapy should be initiated early. Any occlusal adjustments can be performed 6 to 8 weeks postoperatively.

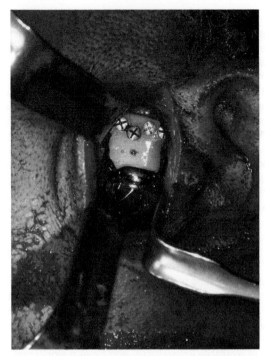

Fig. 13. This patient has undergone total joint replacement. This image shows the new fossa component that has been secured to the zygoma.

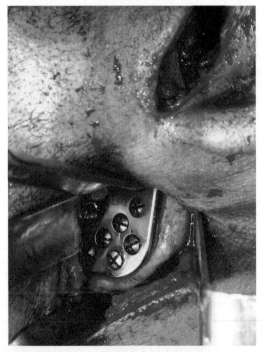

Fig. 14. The ramus component of the total joint is seen here. The component is fixed along posterior ramus and is fixated with multiple screws.

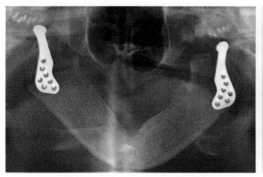 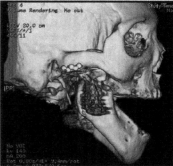

Fig. 15. Panoramic radiograph and 3D rendering of a computed tomography of a patient that has undergone total joint replacement.

Potential complications are numerous and include infection, pain, facial nerve damage, excessive wear of material, malocclusion, and heterotopic bone formation leading to ankylosis. Some surgeons opt to place autogenous fat in the joint space to minimize heterotopic bone formation. Infections are generally reported in 2% to 3% of patients. Wolford and colleagues[30] showed that an infected prosthesis can reasonably be expected to be maintained if the infection is aggressively treated with incision and drainage, placement of irrigating drains, Betadine scrub, and IV antibiotics.

SUMMARY

TMD is a complex group of disorders, and the stage of advancement of the disease determines the recommended treatment. Nonsurgical therapy is first line for early and intermediate cases. Arthrocentesis and arthroscopy are minimally invasive outpatient procedures that are successful in treating Wilkes Class II and III patients. Open-joint surgery is performed on patients who have more advanced disc degeneration or ankylosis. The joint can be instrumented, or the condyle can be removed entirely such as gap arthroplasty. Finally, TJR is reserved for patients with severely limited function and ankylosis. Dental providers should be cognizant of diagnosing and guiding patients to specialists when indicated. A multidisciplinary approach is essential to provide patients with optimal care.

CLINICS CARE POINTS

- Arthrocentesis and arthroscopy are minimally invasive procedures that are effective in improving patient's pain and function.
- Arthroplasty is effective in treating patients with temporomandibular disorders that fail minimally invasive surgery. Various methods of this procedure exist.
- Total joint replacement is highly effective in improving function in patients with ankylosis and severely limited mouth opening.

DISCLOSURE

V.B. Ziccardi serves as consultant for Axogen, Inc., Alachua, Florida. P. Henein has nothing to disclose.

REFERENCES

1. Fonseca RJ. Oral and maxillofacial surgery. Book 2. Section 3. In: Frost DE, editor. 3rd edition. St. Louis, Missouri: Elsevier - Health Sciences Division; 2018. p. 770–940.
2. Wright EF, Klasser GD. Manual of temporomandibular disorders. 4th edition. Ames: Jowa,John Wiley & Sons; 2019.
3. Orofacial Pain: Guidelines for Assessment, Diagnosis, and Management, Fifth Edition. Available at: http://www.quintpub.com/display_detail.php3?psku=B6102#.YfoBK-rMKUk. Accessed February 1, 2022.
4. Bechtold TE, Saunders C, Decker RS, et al. Osteophyte formation and matrix mineralization in a TMJ osteoarthritis mouse model are associated with ectopic hedgehog signaling. Matrix Biol J Int Soc Matrix Biol 2016;52-54:339–54.
5. Nitzan DW, Samson B, Better H. Long-term outcome of arthrocentesis for sudden-onset, persistent, severe closed lock of the temporomandibular joint. J Oral Maxillofac Surg 1997;55(2):151–7.
6. Kaneyama K, Segami N, Nishimura M, et al. The ideal lavage volume for removing bradykinin, interleukin-6, and protein from the temporomandibular joint by arthrocentesis. J Oral Maxillofac Surg 2004;62(6):657–61.
7. Gulen H, Ataoglu H, Haliloglu S, et al. Proinflammatory cytokines in temporomandibular joint synovial fluid before and after arthrocentesis. Oral Surg Oral Med Oral Pathol Oral Radiol Endod 2009;107(5):e1–4.
8. Dolwick MF, Dimitroulis G. A re-evaluation of the importance of disc position in temporomandibular disorders. Aust Dent J 1996;41(3):184–7.
9. Israel HA. The use of arthroscopic surgery for treatment of temporomandibular joint disorders. J Oral Maxillofac Surg 1999;57(5):579–82.
10. Reston JT, Turkelson CM. Meta-analysis of surgical treatments for temporomandibular articular disorders. J Oral Maxillofac Surg 2003;61(1):3–10.
11. McCain JP, Hossameldin RH. Advanced Arthroscopy of the Temporomandibular Joint. Atlas Oral Maxillofac Surg Clin North Am 2011;19(2):145–67.
12. Murakami K. Rationale of arthroscopic surgery of the temporomandibular joint. J Oral Biol Craniofac Res 2013;3(3):126–34.
13. González-García R, Usandizaga JLGD, Rodríguez-Campo FJ. Arthroscopic Anatomy and Lysis and Lavage of the Temporomandibular Joint. Atlas Oral Maxillofac Surg Clin North Am 2011;19(2):131–44.
14. CARTER JB. Complications of TMJ arthroscopy : a review of 2225 cases. Review of the 1988 annual scientific sessions abstract. J Oral Maxillofac Surg 1988;46:M14–5.
15. The case for mandibular condylotomy in the treatment of the painful, deranged temporomandibular joint - ScienceDirect. Available at: https://www.sciencedirect.com/science/article/abs/pii/S0278239197904493. Accessed February 1, 2022.
16. Hall HD. Modification of the modified condylotomy. J Oral Maxillofac Surg 1996;54(5):548–51 [discussion 551-2].
17. Ellis (DDS) E, Zide MF. Surgical approaches to the facial skeleton. Philadelphia, Pennsylvania: Lippincott Williams & Wilkins; 2006. p. 230–3.
18. McCarty WL, Farrar WB. Surgery for internal derangements of the temporomandibular joint. J Prosthet Dent 1979;42(2):191–6.
19. Takaku S, Toyoda T. Long-term evaluation of discectomy of the temporomandibular joint. J Oral Maxillofac Surg 1994;52(7):722–6.

20. Eriksson L, Westesson PL. Long-term evaluation of meniscectomy of the tempo-romandibular joint. J Oral Maxillofac Surg 1985;43(4):263–9.
21. Cavalcanti do Egito Vasconcelos B, Viana Bessa Nogueira R, Vago Cypriano R. Treatment of temporomandibular joint ankylosis by gap arthroplasty. Cavalcanti Egito Vascon Belmiro Viana Bessa Nogueira Ricardo Vago Cypriano Rafael Treat Temporomandibular Jt Ankylosis Gap Arthroplasty En Med Oral Patol Oral Cir Bu-cal Ed Inglesa 11 1 2006 15-. 2006. Available at: https://roderic.uv.es/handle/10550/63577. Accessed February 1, 2022.
22. Roychoudhury A, Parkash H, Trikha A. Functional restoration by gap arthroplasty in temporomandibular joint ankylosis: a report of 50 cases. Oral Surg Oral Med Oral Pathol Oral Radiol Endodontology 1999;87(2):166–9.
23. Williamson RA, McNamara D, McAuliffe W. True eminectomy for internal derange-ment of the temporomandibular joint. Br J Oral Maxillofac Surg 2000;38(5):554–60.
24. Arthroscopic eminoplasty for habitual dislocation of the temporomandibular joint: preliminary study - ScienceDirect. Available at: https://www.sciencedirect.com/science/article/abs/pii/S1010518200900866. Accessed February 1, 2022.
25. Undt G. Temporomandibular Joint Eminectomy for Recurrent Dislocation. Atlas Oral Maxillofac Surg Clin North Am 2011;19(2):189–206.
26. Gruber EA, McCullough J, Sidebottom AJ. Medium-term outcomes and compli-cations after total replacement of the temporomandibular joint. Prospective outcome analysis after 3 and 5 years. Br J Oral Maxillofac Surg 2015;53(5):412–5.
27. Chowdhury SKR, Saxena V, Rajkumar K, et al. Evaluation of Total Alloplastic Temporomandibular Joint Replacement in TMJ Ankylosis. J Maxillofac Oral Surg 2019;18(2):293–8.
28. Perrott DH, Umeda H, Kaban LB. Costochondral graft construction/reconstruc-tion of the ramus/condyle unit: Long-term follow-up. Int J Oral Maxillofac Surg 1994;23(6, Part 1):321–8.
29. Quinn PD, Granquist EJ, editors. Atlas of temporomandibular joint surgery. 2nd edition. Ames, Lowa: John Wiley & Sons Inc; 2015.
30. Wolford LM, Rodrigues DB, McPhillips A. Management of the Infected Temporo-mandibular Joint Total Joint Prosthesis. J Oral Maxillofac Surg 2010;68(11):2810–23.

Temporomandibular Joint Disorders and the Eating Experience

Cibele Nasri-Heir, DDS, MSD[a,b], Riva Touger-Decker, PhD, RD, CDN[c,*]

KEYWORDS

- Temporomandibular joint disorder • Diet • Orofacial pain • Nutrition

KEY POINTS

- Clinicians need to be aware of and sensitive to the impact of the TMD on patients' eating ability, eating experience, ERQOL and appetite.
- Careful attention to patients' eating ability, guidance on positive adaptive eating behaviors, and referrals to an RDN help patients maintain a healthy diet and reduce maladaptive eating behaviors.
- Provide positive adaptive suggestions based on patients' diets and avoid instructing patients to follow a "soft diet."
- Ask patients about how the condition of their mouth has altered their ability to eat, appetite, eating-related quality of life, and diet quality.

INTRODUCTION AND BACKGROUND

The relationship between temporomandibular joint disorders (TMDs) and diet is multidirectional. The Fédération Dentaire Internationale (FDI) World Dental Federation defines oral health as "multifaceted and includes the ability to speak, smile, smell, taste, touch, chew, swallow and convey a wide range of emotions through facial expressions with confidence and without pain, discomfort, and disease of the craniofacial complex (FDI)."[1] Individuals with TMD have compromised oral health by virtue of the influence of the disease on masticatory function and the ability to swallow and sometimes smile and speak without pain or discomfort. As part of the stomatognathic system, the temporomandibular joint (TMJ) works closely with other components of

[a] Department of Diagnostic Sciences, Center for Temporomandibular Disorders and Orofacial Pain, Rutgers School of Dental Medicine, 110 Bergen Street, Newark, NJ 07101, USA; [b] Department of Diagnostic Sciences, Rutgers School of Dental Medicine, Rutgers, The State University, 110, Bergen Street, Room D-867, Newark, NJ 07101-1709, USA; [c] Department of Diagnostic Sciences, Rutgers School of Dental Medicine, Rutgers School of Health Professions, 110 Bergen Street, Newark, NJ 07101, USA
* Corresponding author.
E-mail address: decker@rutgers.edu

Dent Clin N Am 67 (2023) 367–377
https://doi.org/10.1016/j.cden.2022.11.005
0011-8532/23/© 2022 Elsevier Inc. All rights reserved.

that system, particularly the muscles and teeth, to facilitate mandibular opening, biting, chewing, and swallowing.

TMD pathophysiology remains unknown and has created controversy over the years; evidence suggests that biological, psychological, and social factors combine to predispose, initiate, or perpetuate painful TMD.[2] It is a complex disorder with multiple causes consistent with a biopsychosocial model of illness.[3,4] The term TMD encompasses a group of painful and nonpainful musculoskeletal conditions that involve the TMJs, the masticatory muscles, and all associated tissues.[2,5] The most common types of TMDs are myogenous, or muscle-generated pain and arthrogenous or joint-generated pain.[6] Myalgia affects around 80% of patients with TMD and is the most common TMD diagnosis along with arthralgia, which frequently occurs together with myalgia.[7,8] The Diagnostic Criteria/Temporomandibular Disorder (DC/TMD) also includes headache attributed to TMDs, which is a headache that occurs in the temporal region secondary to painful TMD and that is aggravated by jaw movement, jaw function, or parafunction.[9] All other possible headache diagnoses should be ruled out before attributing the headache to the TMD diagnosis. Other common types of TMD include primary disc displacement and degenerative diseases. The 3 main signs and symptoms of TMD are pain, limited range of mandibular movement, and TMJ sounds that are most frequently described as "popping," "clicking," grating, or crepitus.[2] Pain is often the main complaint affecting the muscles of mastication and the periauricular area, and it is aggravated or provoked by chewing and other mandibular activities such as yawning or talking.[4]

The musculoskeletal nature of the disorder, the associated pain, and treatments can influence appetite and mechanical factors involved with eating, drinking, and swallowing, thus affecting dietary intake and, potentially, nutritional status. Oral function challenges, along with the emotional and social impacts of the disease on activities of daily living and eating-related quality of life (ERQOL), are common and can affect food choices as well as diet quality and composition.

Management of TMD requires a patient-centered interprofessional team approach, including orofacial pain specialists, physical therapists, registered dietitian nutritionists (RDNs), and other health professionals.[10] The interprofessional collaboration of the orofacial pain specialist, RDN and physical therapist can help the patient improve their ability to eat and thus positively affect their ERQOL and nutrition status. This article will review the evidence regarding the impact of TMD on functional ability to eat comfortably, ERQOL and nutrition status, and address dietary management approaches.

DISCUSSION

There is a paucity of scientifically sound research on TMD, dietary approaches to management, and nutrition status. Earlier research has explored TMD symptoms affecting eating ability,[11–14] dysphagia risk,[15–18] and dietary interventions with vitamin D[19] or a gluten-free diet.[20] However, there are no evidence-based dietary guidelines for patients with TMD, despite the profound impact this chronic disease can have on masticatory function and ERQOL.[21]

Therapies Used to Treat Temporomandibular Joint Disorder

Conservative therapies are the first-line treatment of TMD, including patient education, self-care techniques, intraoral appliances, physical therapy and acupuncture, biobehavioral therapy, and pharmacotherapy.[2,21] Pharmacologic treatments range from simple analgesic medications to neuromodulatory agents, usually combined with other therapy modalities.[4]

The most commonly used pharmacologic agents for the management of TMDs include analgesics, nonsteroidal anti-inflammatory drugs (NSAIDs), corticosteroids, benzodiazepines, muscle relaxants, and low-dose antidepressants.[2,22] The analgesics (nonopiate preparations), corticosteroids, and benzodiazepines are indicated for acute TMD pain; NSAIDs and muscle relaxants may be used for both acute and chronic conditions.[2] Neuromodulatory agents such as tricyclic antidepressants (TCAs), serotonin-noradrenaline reuptake inhibitors (SSRIs), and gabapentin are used to treat chronic TMD.[4,23]

The clinician should be aware of and inform patients of the potential adverse effects and medication–medication and medication–supplement interactions that may occur. Unintentional weight gain and xerostomia are common adverse reactions to SSRIs, TCAs, and cyclobenzaprine that patients should be cautioned about.[24] Gastrointestinal side effects ranging from gastrointestinal distress to altered bowel function and changes in taste have been reported with benzodiazepines.[24] There are gastrointestinal side effects of NSAIDs, including dyspepsia and gastric and duodenal ulcers.[25] Although the medications may help TMD-associated pain, their impact on appetite and eating should be considered when counseling patients.

Impact of Temporomandibular Joint Disorder on the Eating Experience, Weight, and Symptoms of Dysphagia

As a chronic condition, the impact of TMD on eating ability and diet is long-term. Recent research on the impact of TMD on masticatory function and swallowing has demonstrated the breadth and depth of its effect on all aspects of eating, including appetite, food preparation, biting, chewing and swallowing, and ERQOL.[11,13,14,16] Ferreira and colleagues[12] explored chewing difficulties in adults (aged 18–41 years) in Italy. The investigators found that in these adults with TMD, chewing behaviors and eating patterns were negatively affected compared with those without TMD. Edwards and colleagues[11] surveyed adults with TMD who volunteered to complete a survey and 3-day food diary and found that participants with a limited mandibular opening (self-reported) had more pain, had fewer foods they could eat, experienced reduced enjoyment of food, modified their approach to food preparation, and lost weight. Participants reported boiling, pureeing, and mashing foods to create a soft diet. Those who modified their food preparation consumed less dietary fiber than those who did not. There were no other significant differences in energy or nutrient intake; however, the sample size of participants who completed the 3-day diaries was small. Gilheany and colleagues explored masticatory and swallowing difficulties using a subjective questionnaire in an Irish cohort of 178 adults with TMD. In this sample of adults with TMD, 90% reported masticatory pain, 78% reported fatigue with mastication, 26% reported weight loss due to difficulty with eating and drinking, and one-third reported difficulty swallowing. Participants also experienced difficulty chewing hard and sometimes soft foods.[16]

Although dysphagia may not be typically associated with TMD, individuals with TMD may experience symptoms of oral dysphagia, which involves factors affecting the first or oral phase of swallowing.[26] Oral phase symptoms include limited mandibular movement, drooling, poor tongue movement, inability to form a seal with the lips, difficulty chewing, and difficulty initiating a swallow. Prolonged eating time and fatigue with eating are also signs of dysphagia. Although limited, there is a body of evidence exploring the relationships between TMD and symptoms of oral dysphagia.[15,16,18] Gilheany and colleagues found that self-reported symptoms of oral dysphagia reported by participants were related to mastication, oromotor function (including slurred or painful speech, bruxism), pain, hearing, and psychosocial factors.[16] About 99% of the sample had one or more problems with eating, drinking, or swallowing. Although this was a single study in Ireland, the results are consistent with other studies regarding masticatory difficulties and weight changes and provide insight into the added problem of dysphagia faced by individuals with TMD. Others[18] have also reported weaker tongue protrusion and swallowing strength and greater chewing difficulty in adults with TMD compared with controls. A systematic review on the topic[15] similarly identified symptoms of oral dysphagia in adults with TMD. It also supported prior research regarding difficult and painful mastication, prolonged eating time, and fatigue from chewing, all of which may be symptoms of dysphagia.

These eating-related symptoms also contribute to the symptom burden experienced by patients with orofacial pain and the negative impacts on ERQOL. Symptom burden is "the subjective, quantifiable prevalence, frequency, and severity of symptoms placing a physiologic burden on patients and producing multiple negative, physical and emotional patient responses."[27] Given the considerable impact TMD has on the ability to eat, and ERQOL, consideration of the symptom burden patients with this disease experience can provide meaningful insights to the clinician when approaching disease management with the patient. Safour and colleagues[14] investigated the eating experience of adults with TMD using a phenomenological approach with adults aged 25 to 51 years in Montreal, Canada. ERQOL was negatively impacted due to chewing difficulties, constantly feeling bloated, and changing diets dramatically due to their TMD. Meals took much longer to eat, and favorite foods could no longer be eaten. Participants also reported systemic impacts of TMD, including constipation and bloating, due to the changes they had to make in their diets. Weight changes (both gain and loss) were common; patients with weight loss ate less because of jaw pain.

Risk of Malnutrition in Adults with Temporomandibular Joint Disorder

Risk factors for malnutrition, including micronutrient deficiencies in adults with TMD, include difficulty eating and swallowing, weight loss, and poor diet. Unintentional weight loss of greater than 10% in 6 months or less reflects a risk for malnutrition. Patients with TMD who experience weight loss should be probed for reasons behind the weight loss to determine if it is due to an inadequate diet or a systemic condition. Referrals to a RDN for a comprehensive nutrition assessment and medical nutrition therapy are warranted; if a systemic condition is suspected, the patient should also be referred to their primary care provider.

Adults with TMD may risk micronutrient deficiencies due to maladaptive eating behaviors and nutritionally inadequate diets. The research in this area is dated,[28] limited to single institutions in a country,[29,30,] and heterogeneous. In a sample of patients with TMD in Texas, USA, who had implant surgery, Mehra and Wolford[28] found that one-third or more of the patients had micronutrient deficiencies evidenced by low serum levels of iron, beta-carotene, vitamins B1, B6, B12, C, ferritin and folate, and clinically apparent glossitis, cheilosis, hair loss, and anemia. Almost a decade later, in Saudi Arabia, Ahmed and colleagues examined adults with TMD for clinical and biochemical signs of micronutrient deficiencies and also found that one-third or more had low serum values for vitamins D and C, iron, and "B-complex" with clinical symptoms similar to Mehra and Wolford.[30] In contrast, a more recent study by Staniszewski and colleagues[29] found no evidence of micronutrient deficiencies based on biochemical assays in a population of adults with TMD in Norway. The limitations of and potential for heterogeneity among studies is beyond the scope of this article; however, because patients with TMD often take dietary supplements, it could be that while they are missing the food sources of these nutrients in their diets, they are getting them through supplements. Although dietary supplements may provide micronutrients essential for health, they do not provide the other properties found in the foods such as fruits, vegetables, and whole grains, which are also essential for health.

Diet and Nutrition Risk Evaluation and Management of Patients with Temporomandibular Joint Disorder

Before any dietary guidance can be provided to patients, it is essential to assess each individual in regard to the symptom burdens they are experiencing related to diet, their ERQOL, weight and weight history, current dietary patterns, and how their TMD symptoms affect when, what, where, and how they eat. Responses will provide insight into adaptive and maladaptive behaviors and the extent of the impact of the TMD on their nutrition status. **Table 1**[31] provides a sample interview guide that any clinician can use to assess TMD symptoms in relation to their diet and ERQOL. Asking such questions early in the patient evaluation process can help identify patients needing referrals to other health professionals. The medical and dental history and list of patient medications are also important to fully assess patient risks and intervention needs. The use of dietary supplements should be carefully evaluated relative to medications the patient is taking to determine any possible medication–nutrient interactions. Although more than 50% of US adults use dietary supplements, there is a paucity of scientifically sound evidence of any benefits from specific dietary supplements for TMD.

Questions about whether patients fear that eating will cause pain and how they have modified their food and fluid consumption can provide insight into positive adaptive and maladaptive behaviors. Responses to questions about weight change, problems with constipation, bloating, and avoidance of major food groups or fad diets can be used to determine if the patient needs to be referred to an RDN for medical nutrition therapy. Some patient symptoms may be related to self-imposed diet changes. A diet low in fiber due to avoidance of whole grains, fruits, and vegetables can contribute to constipation and bloating and place the patient at risk for micronutrient deficiencies. Although oral health-care professionals can provide tailored guidance on a diet for TMD, patients with unintentional weight gain or loss, poor appetite, constipation, or bloating related to their TMD, maladaptive dietary behaviors, or who are avoiding many foods and food groups because of their TMD should be referred to an RDN for a comprehensive nutrition assessment and individualized medical nutrition therapy. Patients with symptoms of dysphagia or who complain of swallowing difficulties should be referred to a speech and language pathologist for evaluation.

Diet Modifications for Temporomandibular Joint Disorder

With the lack of consensus on dietary management for TMD, patients may eliminate whole food groups such as whole grains, fruits, and vegetables because of difficulty or pain with biting, chewing, or swallowing. Clinicians similarly lack the resources to guide patients on an approach to eating with TMD. Vitamin D supplements and a gluten-free diet have been proposed as adjunctive treatment strategies.[19,20] Although it is beyond the scope of this article to discuss the theories behind the potential association between TMD and either a gluten-free diet or additional vitamin D, there's a dearth of scientifically sound evidence to support either association.

A soft diet is commonly recommended for individuals with TMD.[21,32,33] The term itself is open to wide interpretation by clinicians and consumers. Soft breads and rolls require a more significant masticatory effort than popcorn, broken thin pretzel sticks, and whole grains such as brown rice, wheat berries, or couscous. Chopped tomato and other chopped or minced vegetable salads are more appealing, contain more nutrients than boiled and pureed vegetables, and may actually require less masticatory effort than a soft diet. A soft diet can lead to reductions in fruit, vegetable, and whole

Table 1
Diet and nutrition risk for temporomandibular joint disorder interview guide for clinicians

Question	Recommended Actions for YES Responses
Have you altered what you eat and drink because of your TMD?	Probe by asking: Please describe what you have changed in your food and drink choices and the duration of these changes This will help the provider tailor future advice Do you now avoid eating or drinking anything in particular because of your TMD? If yes, what? Are there favorite foods or beverages you are now avoiding because of your TMD? Would you want to add these foods back if there were ways to do so that would not cause pain? A positive response reflects a patient's willingness to develop adaptive behaviors
Is it difficult or painful to open your mouth, bite, chew, or swallow?	Please tell me what is painful and what is difficult Peeling, cutting, and chopping food can make eating easier and less painful Limiting sticky foods such as peanut or almond butter can help to avoid painful eating
Are you avoiding any specific food groups such as fresh fruits, and vegetables, whole grain bread, nuts, and others because of TMD?	Fruits and vegetables: peel fruits and vegetables with skin and chop, mince, or mash. If needed, cooking vegetables such as squash, carrots, broccoli, and cauliflower until tender before cutting may also help to reduce painful eating Toasting and slicing whole grain bread into thin slices may make them easier to eat than soft white bread Break thin pretzel sticks and other thin crackers into small pieces to reduce the need to open the mouth wide and minimize biting and chewing Chop nuts finely and add to hot cereals, yogurt, or puddings Make chopped fruit or vegetable salads Use your knife and fork as your "teeth" to cut foods into small pieces to minimize biting and chewing needed Make a smoothie
Are you avoiding going out for meals or eating with others because of your TMD?	If yes: What specifically do you avoid? Try restaurants where foods may be served cut, chopped, or pureed such as Asian, Middle Eastern, or Indian restaurants, those specializing in soups or places you can ask to have your food specially ordered

(continued on next page)

Table 1 (continued)	
Question	**Recommended Actions for YES Responses**
How has your weight changed? If unsure tell me if your waistlines feel tight or loose (hint 10 lbs = 1 clothing size)	If unintentional weight loss is revealed: encourage the patient to see their physician and a registered dietitian nutritionist for medical nutrition therapy If unintentional weight gain is revealed: suggest that they may want to seek the counseling of a registered dietitian nutritionist for medical nutrition therapy to avoid unintentional weight gain and improve diet quality
Are you taking any vitamin, mineral, herbal, or other dietary supplements?	If yes, probe by asking: What do you take, how often, how much and why? Probe further by asking if the supplement does what they thought it would do. Decision support tools and databases such as *Lexicomp* and Natural *Medicines Database* can be used to evaluate risks of interactions, side effects and potential benefits
Are you following or have you tried any special diet because of your TMD?	Probe to find out what diet, rationale for following it and whether they think it is working
Do you ever experience constipation?	If yes: Is this new since you were diagnosed with TMD? Do you think it is due to your changes in diet? How are you managing it?
Do you ever experience bloating before, during, or after a meal?	If yes: What do you think is causing it? (Probe to determine if its related to their diet or constipation)
Does it take you the same, more, or less time to eat a meal or snack since you were diagnosed with TMD?	If yes: Probe to understand why.

Adapted from: Nasri-Heir C, Epstein JB, Touger-Decker R, Benoliel R. What should we tell patients with painful temporomandibular disorders about what to eat? *Journal of the American Dental Association*. 2016;147(8):667-71.

grain intake and a resultant drop in dietary fiber and micronutrient intake. The goal of dietary guidance for individuals with TMD should be to mechanically alter the food forms to accommodate patients' limited mandibular opening and minimize the amount of biting and chewing needed.[31,33] "Clinicians can advise patients to use their knives and forks as they might their teeth, consciously cutting foods into small pieces, as well as provide recommendations on how to modify food selections to reduce mandibular workload and minimize jaw pain."[31] The goal of dietary guidance is to maximize diet quality and ERQOL and avoid or limit painful eating.

Table 2[31] provides recommendations to share with patients to help them modify their diet and maximize nutrient intake while reducing the mandibular workload.

Table 2
Guide to food choices and preparation hints for individuals with temporomandibular joint disorder

Overall Principles

- Cut all foods well
- Use gravies or sauces to moisten foods to a comfortable consistency
- Peel and chop fruits and vegetables with skins (except for berries)
- Chop whole foods to consistencies that are comfortable to eat
- Take small bites of food
- Choose foods from all food groups for healthy food choices
- Leave sufficient time to eat
- Peel, chop, shred and mince foods to a consistency that is easy to eat
- Use sauces, gravies, natural vegetable and fruit juices, and broths to moisten foods and add flavor
- At the table, use a knife and fork to cut food as needed

Food Group	Food Options and Preparation Hints
Fruits	Peel all fruits with hard/chewy skin: such as apples, peaches, plums, pears Chop: whole (peeled) fruits Use a blender to turn fruits into smoothies or sauces Make smoothies with any peeled fruits in a blender, adding dairy or nondairy milks or yogurts
Vegetables	Greens such as spinach, chard, kale, collards: wash, steam, or cook for 2–3 min and chop fine into ribbon-like thickness Tomatoes: chop Cucumbers: peel and chop fine Root vegetables like carrots, parsnips, beets: Peel and either shred or chop/mince fine (if chopped, cook after chopping) Other vegetables: cook until tender, chop Potatoes (white or sweet): cook, chop, or mash Make smoothies or juices with vegetables in a blender Chop vegetables and mix with water or broth and cook to make soups
Legumes, seeds, and nuts	Legumes should be cooked, and those larger than a pea should be mashed or pureed Chop nuts or use nut or seed butters
Animal and other protein foods	Poultry/meats: Cook until tender, moisten with broth, gravies, or other sauces and cut into bite-size pieces Fish: cook and cut into bite-size pieces or shred, soften with sauces as desired, or chop and mix into a fish salad Tofu, tempeh—Chop to bite-size pieces; tempeh may need moistening
Dairy/lactose free dairy alternatives	All milk products, yogurts, and cheeses as tolerated
Bread, cereals, grains	Hot or cold cereals (hint: soften cereal in milk) Couscous, quinoa, farro, rice, and other cooked grains Orzo and other small pasta cooked until tender Thinly slice whole grain bread and rolls, toast, and cut into small pieces Thin crackers broken into small pieces

Note: The extent to which foods may be cut, chopped, minced, or pureed varies based on what you can do comfortably. The guidelines are intended to help you select healthful and preferred foods and enjoy eating whether at home or out of the home.

Adapted from: Nasri-Heir C, Epstein JB, Touger-Decker R, Benoliel R. What should we tell patients with painful temporomandibular disorders about what to eat? Journal of the American Dental Association. 2016;147(8):667-71.

Patient-centered care is essential to maximize nutritional well-being; dietary guidance by oral health professionals should be individualized to each patient's functional limitations and challenges with the eating experience. The primary goals should be to encourage positive adaptive behaviors, help the patient eat comfortably, and reduce the symptom burden experienced by the patient. Working toward these goals can also reduce the risk of unintentional weight gain or loss and micronutrient deficiencies and address some of the systemic symptoms of TMD such as bloating and constipation. Targeting recommendations to address each patient's functional limitations due to their TMD can help improve their appetite and functional ability to eat and ERQOL. Diet quality and adequacy can also be achieved if the patient can be helped to adapt their diet to eat comfortably. The guidelines and tips in **Table 2** can be applied to patients' socioeconomic circumstances and cultural or religious preferences.

SUMMARY

Management of adults with TMD requires an interprofessional approach. Clinicians need to be aware of and sensitive to the impact of the TMD on patients' eating ability, eating experience, ERQOL, and appetite. Oral health professionals can collaborate with RDNs and other health professionals to improve patient outcomes. Many of the symptoms of TMD affect an individual's mandibular opening and ability to bite, chew, and swallow food. Careful attention to the patient's symptoms relative to eating ability, guidance on modifying the diet with positive adaptive behaviors, and referrals to an RDN may help patients maintain a healthy diet and reduce weight loss and maladaptive eating behaviors. Further research is required to develop evidence-based guidelines for the diet management of patients with TMD.

CLINICS CARE POINTS

- Determine if and how TMD has affected patients' abilities to open their mouths, bite, chew, and swallow.
- Ask patients about how the condition of their mouth has altered their ability to eat, appetite, ERQOL, and diet quality.
- Provide positive adaptive suggestions based on patients' diet and avoid instructing patients to follow a "soft diet."
- Screen patients for weight loss and maladaptive eating behaviors.
- Provide dietary guidance individualized to the patient's symptoms and lifestyle.
- Refer patients with weight loss, decreased appetite, or difficulty meeting their nutrient needs to an RDN.

DISCLOSURE

The authors have nothing to disclose.

REFERENCES

1. FDI World Dental Federation. FDI's definition of oral health. Available at: http://www.fdiworlddental.org/fdis-definition-oral-health. Accessed August 8th 2022.
2. American Academy of Orofacial Pain (AAOP). Differential Diagnosis and Management of TMDs. In: Leeuw Rd, Klasser GD, editors. Orofacial pain : guidelines

for assessment, diagnosis, and management. 6th edition. Hanover Park, IL: Quintessence Publishing Co, Inc.; 2018. p. 143–60.

3. Slade GD, Fillingim RB, Sanders AE, et al. Summary of findings from the OPPERA prospective cohort study of incidence of first-onset temporomandibular disorder: implications and future directions. J Pain Dec 2013;14(12 Suppl):T116–24.

4. Palmer J, Durham J. Temporomandibular disorders. BJA education 2021;21(2): 44–50.

5. Greene CS. Managing the care of patients with temporomandibular disorders: a new guideline for care. J Am Dental Assoc (1939) 2010;141(9):1086–8.

6. Nitzan D, Heir GM, Dolwick F, et al. Pain and dysfunction of the temporomandibular joint. In: Sharav Y, Benoliel R, editors. *Orofacial Pain and Headache*. 2nd edition. Batavia, IL: Quintessence Publishing Co, Inc; 2015. p. 257–318.

7. List T, Dworkin SF. Comparing TMD diagnoses and clinical findings at Swedish and US TMD centers using research diagnostic criteria for temporomandibular disorders. Journal of Orofacial Pain 1996;10(3):240–53.

8. List T, Jensen RH. Temporomandibular disorders: Old ideas and new concepts. Cephalalgia : Int J Headache Jun 2017;37(7):692–704.

9. Schiffman E, Ohrbach R, Truelove E, et al. Diagnostic Criteria for Temporomandibular Disorders (DC/TMD) for Clinical and Research Applications: recommendations of the International RDC/TMD Consortium Network* and Orofacial Pain Special Interest Group. J Oral Facial Pain Headache 2014;28(1):6–27.

10. Ohrbach R, Greene C. Temporomandibular Disorders: Priorities for Research and Care. J Dental Res Jul 2022;101(7):742–3.

11. Edwards DC, Bowes CC, Penlington C, et al. Temporomandibular disorders and dietary changes: A cross-sectional survey. J Oral Rehabil Aug 2021;48(8):873–9.

12. Ferreira CLP, Sforza C, Rusconi FME, et al. Masticatory behaviour and chewing difficulties in young adults with temporomandibular disorders. J Oral Rehabil Jun 2019;46(6):533–40.

13. Ferreira MC, Porto de Toledo I, Dutra KL, et al. Association between chewing dysfunctions and temporomandibular disorders: A systematic review. J Oral Rehabil Oct 2018;45(10):819–35.

14. Safour W, Hovey R. A phenomenologic study about the dietary habits and digestive complications for people living with temporomandibular joint disorder. J Oral Facial Pain Headache 2019;3(4):377–88.

15. Gilheaney Ó, Béchet S, Kerr P, et al. The prevalence of oral stage dysphagia in adults presenting with temporomandibular disorders: a systematic review and meta-analysis. Acta odontologica Scand 2018;76(6):448–58.

16. Gilheaney Ó, Stassen LF, Walshe M. Prevalence, Nature, and Management of Oral Stage Dysphagia in Adults With Temporomandibular Joint Disorders: Findings From an Irish Cohort. J Oral Maxill Surg 2018;76(8):1665–76.

17. Marim GC, Machado BCZ, Trawitzki LVV, et al. Tongue strength, masticatory and swallowing dysfunction in patients with chronic temporomandibular disorder. Physiol Behav Oct 15 2019;210:112616.

18. Rosa RR, Bueno M, Migliorucci RR, et al. Tongue function and swallowing in individuals with temporomandibular disorders. J Appl Oral Sci : revista FOB 2020;28:e20190355.

19. Kui A, Buduru S, Labunet A, et al. Vitamin D and Temporomandibular Disorders: What Do We Know So Far? Nutrients 2021;13(4).

20. Araújo Oliveira Buosi J, Abreu Nogueira SM, Sousa MP, et al. Gluten-Free Diet Reduces Pain in Women with Myofascial Pain in Masticatory Muscles: A

Preliminary Randomized Controlled Trial. J Oral Facial Pain Headache 2021; 35(3):199–207.

21. National academies of sciences engineering, medicine. Temporomandibular disorders: priorities for research and care. Washington, DC: The National Academies Press; 2020.

22. Dionne RA. Pharmacologic treatments for temporomandibular disorders. Oral Surgery,Oral Medicine, Oral Pathology, Oral Radiology, and Endodontics 1997; 83(1):134–42.

23. Haviv Y, Rettman A, Aframian D, et al. Myofascial pain: an open study on the pharmacotherapeutic response to stepped treatment with tricyclic antidepressants and gabapentin. J Oral Facial Pain Headache 2015;29(2):144–51.

24. Lexicomp. Available at: https://online.lexi.com/lco/action/home. Accessed August 8, 2022 through Rutgers University Library.

25. Scheiman JM. NSAID-induced Gastrointestinal Injury: A Focused Update for Clinicians. J Clin Gastroenterol 2016;50(1):5–10.

26. Wieseke A, Bantz D, Siktberg L, et al. Assessment and early diagnosis of dysphagia. Geriatr Nurs (New York, N.Y.) 2008;29(6):376–83.

27. Gapstur RL. Symptom burden: a concept analysis and implications for oncology nurses. Oncol Nurs Forum 2007;34(3):673–80.

28. Mehra P, Wolford LM. Serum nutrient deficiencies in the patient with complex temporomandibular joint problems. Proceedings (Baylor University. Medical Center) 2008;21(3):243–7.

29. Staniszewski K, Lygre H, Berge T, et al. Serum Analysis in Patients with Temporomandibular Disorders: A Controlled Cross-Sectional Study in Norway. Pain Res Manag 2019;2019:1360725.

30. Ahmed S, Tabassum N, Al Dayel O, et al. Nutritional assessment in temporomandibular disease: Creating awareness on sytemic impact of temporomandibular disorder in Saudi population. J Int Health 2016;8(11):1023–5.

31. Nasri-Heir C, Epstein JB, Touger-Decker R, et al. What should we tell patients with painful temporomandibular disorders about what to eat? J Am Dental Assoc (1939) 2016;147(8):667–71.

32. The TMJ Association. What and How You Eat Matters. Available at: https://tmj.org/living-with-tmj/self-care/. Accessed August 8th, 2022.

33. Durham J, Touger-Decker R, Nixdorf DR, et al. Oro-facial pain and nutrition: a forgotten relationship? J Oral Rehabil 2015;42(1):75–80.

Temporomandibular Joint Disorder Comorbidities

Davis C. Thomas, BDS, DDS, MSD, MSc Med, MSc[a,b,*], Junad Khan, MSD, MPH, PhD[c],
Daniele Manfredini, DDS, PhD[d], Jessica Ailani, MD, FAHS[e]

KEYWORDS

- Temporomandibular joint disorder • Temporomandibular joint • Comorbidities
- Headaches

KEY POINTS

- The comorbidities that affect temporomandibular joint disorder (TMD) pain are crucial for the treating physician to bring about effective management of TMD pain.
- In the absence of delineation of the comorbidities that may condition the patient's experience of TMD pain, the clinician-patient team may most likely encounter the problem of suboptimal management of pain.
- A complete discussion of the numerous comorbidities that affect TMD pain experience is beyond the scope of any manuscript. It is up to pain education programs and individual clinicians to educate the medical community regarding the significance of managing TMD pain through effective management of the comorbidities.
- The discovery of comorbidities in a patient suffering from TMD and TMD pain may necessitate a multidisciplinary approach of management involving more than 1 medical specialty.
- Any clinician attempting to manage TMD and TMD pain must be familiar with the possibility of one or more comorbidities that may profoundly affect the patient's experience of pain.

INTRODUCTION

Comorbidity is largely defined in medical literature as a specific additional condition that exists as temporally related to the condition being explored.[1,2] Temporomandibular joint disorders (TMDs) have been shown to have associations with several comorbidities,

[a] Department of Diagnostic Sciences, Rutgers School of Dental Medicine, 110 Bergen Street, Newark, NJ 07103, USA; [b] Eastman Institute of Oral Health, Rochester, NY, USA; [c] Department of Orofacial Pain and TMJ Disorders, Eastman Institute for Oral Health, 2400 South Clinton Avenue, Building H, Suite #125, Rochester, NY 14618, USA; [d] Department of Biomedical Technologies, School of Dentistry, University of Siena, Viale Bracci - 53100 Siena, Italy; [e] Georgetown Headache Center, Strategic Planning Neurology, Medstar Georgetown University Hospital 3800 Reservoir Road. NW, Washington, DC 20007, USA
* Corresponding author.
E-mail address: davisct1@gmail.com

Dent Clin N Am 67 (2023) 379–392
https://doi.org/10.1016/j.cden.2022.10.005
0011-8532/23/© 2022 Elsevier Inc. All rights reserved.

including, but not limited to, headaches, hypermobility syndromes, fibromyalgia, anxiety/depression, and sleep disorders. Some of the comorbidities, such as hypermobility syndromes, may have a predisposition to many of the TMD symptoms. A sound knowledge about these comorbidities may be crucial in executing the best management modalities for TMDs. For example, management of TMDs using an antidepressant drug such as low-dose amitriptyline may inherently help in the management of comorbid anxiety, depression, and fibromyalgia (FM). Screening for possible comorbidities such as anxiety/depression and sleep disorders may even prove to be a lifesaver for these patients. A TMD patient being screened for the possibility of a systemic factor such as anemia, vitamin deficiencies, nutritional deficiencies, or lack of sleep, may be instrumental in shedding light on the factors conditioning the experience of TMD pain. It must be noted that, because of the multitude of comorbidities that can probably associate with TMD, a comprehensive discussion of the topics is beyond the purview of a single article. The authors encourage readers to refer to the cited articles for additional information. A recent systematic review showed a significant association of comorbid other chronic pain conditions among patients who were diagnosed with TMD.[3] These included chronic migraine, fibromyalgia, and myofascial syndrome.

HEADACHES

Patients who have been diagnosed with TMD are more likely to have associated chronic pain disorders such as chronic migraine, inflammatory bowel syndrome (IBS), FM, and myofascial pain.[3–6] Chronic migraine appears to be 8 times more common in patients diagnosed with TMDs than in the general population.[3,7,8] The Orofacial Pain Prospective Evaluation and Risk Assessment study found that headache was a more common symptom in patients with a painful TMD compared with other chronic overlapping pain conditions such as FM, IBS, and low back pain.[3,5,9,10] Studies have found a positive correlation between painful TMD and migraine, but not between TMD and probable tension type headache (TTH) 30936004.[7] However, other studies have shown an association between TMD and TTH.[11,12] Headaches in general, and migraine in particular, have shown to indicate a higher likelihood of developing TMD. The prevalence and frequency of headaches increase over time in patients who develop TMD.[11] Migraine is widespread in TMD patients with a prevalence/incidence rate of approximately 25% to 50%,[10,13–15] and it is linked to greater physical and psychosocial distress.[13,16–19]

Migraine is common in women between the ages of 20 to 40, and involves activation of the trigeminal nerve, which triggers pain, along with a host of associated symptoms.[20] TMD is also a common disabling disorder seen more often in women between the ages of 20 to 40, involving the activation of the trigeminal nerve and frequently comorbid with primary headache disorders.[21] Migraine patients have approximately 8 times the risk of developing severe TMD as patients without migraine as a comorbidity.[13,14,22] Moreover, there is an association between headache frequency and the duration and intensity of TMD pain.[13,23] Migraine patients with TMDs show more central sensitization symptoms than those without TMD.[24] The central sensitization in migraine can be explained by (among others) the action of calcitonin gene-related peptide (CGRP).[7,25]

Headache secondary to TMD is not well described in the literature,[21] and is considered a secondary headache disorder.[26] The International Classification of Headache Disorders (ICHD3) defines headache attributed to TMD as only rarely occurring as a sole feature of TMD. The full criteria are listed in **Box 1**. The overall prevalence of headache in the TMD population is approximately 60%, with migraine being the most

---

Box 1
International Classification of Headache Disorders Criteria for headache attributed to temporomandibular joint disorders

A. Any headache fulfilling criteria

B. Clinical evidence of a painful pathologic process affecting elements of the temporomandibular joint(s), muscles of mastication, and/or associated structures on one or both sides

C. Evidence of causation demonstrated by at least 2 of the following:
   1. The headache has developed in temporal relation to the onset of the temporomandibular disorder, or led to its discovery
   2. The headache is aggravated by jaw motion, jaw function (eg, chewing) and/or jaw parafunction (eg, bruxism)
   3. The headache is provoked on physical examination by temporalis muscle palpation and/or passive movement of the jaw
   4. Usually temporally located (one or both sides)

D. Not better accounted for by another ICHD-3 diagnosis

---

common, affecting approximately 40% of the people. The second most common associated headache is tension-type headache (approximately 19%).[27–30] The prevalence of TMD in the headache population based on a meta-analysis of published studies was 59.42%.[31] Those with painful-TMD had a higher prevalence of headache at 82.80%, again with migraine being the more common headache. TMD is common in those with primary headache disorders, especially migraine and TTH. People with TMD are twice as likely to have chronic daily headaches with or without migraine.[31] The more severe the TMD, the more severe the migraine[31]

Having both TMD and migraine leads to a significantly greater disability; therefore effective treatment should focus on treating both disorders when they are present.[20] Treating TMD and migraine simultaneously can also improve the therapeutic response for each individual disorder.[21] A multidisciplinary approach is often best in these patient groups. Treatment of TMD starts with patient education and conservative measures. Rest of the jaw and avoiding eating hard, chewy foods, or chewing gum are important. Management of concomitant clenching and grinding should be discussed with patients with TMD as well.[20] Physical therapy is a simple, noninvasive option that can be added to education as a first-line treatment for patients with TMD. Heat or ice to the painful area, self-massage, and range-of-motion exercises can all reduce pain and improve function.[32] If this is only partially effective, a course of physical therapy for active relaxation exercises, passive stretching, deep massage, ultrasound and acupressure, electrical stimulation, transcutaneous electrical nerve stimulation, and myofascial release have been shown to be effective.[33] Jaw appliances, known as splints, night guards, bite guards, or stabilization appliances, have shown some evidence to be helpful when used appropriately in people with TMD. A systematic review has shown good evidence for single-arch, hard, full-coverage stabilization appliances for the treatment of TMD pain.[34] When adjusted properly, these can have a modest effect in the treatment of pain. When splints are used inappropriately, they can cause complications such as misalignment of teeth and occlusal alterations.[20] As stress and anxiety can trigger or worsen TMD, addressing the psychological impact of pain can improve outcomes.[35] There are many ways this can be addressed. Cognitive behavioral therapy can improve anxiety and can be done in person, via telehealth, or using pain psychology-specific applications. If TMD pain continues despite conservative measures, medications can be added to improve symptoms. Oral medications for

TMD pain include nonsteroidal anti-inflammatory drugs (NSAIDs), muscle relaxants, and tricyclic antidepressants in cases of chronic disease and in those with associated headache.[20] Medications should be used for a prescribed interval of time and not indefinitely to avoid adverse events.[20] Medications employed to manage headaches (including NSAIDs and beta blockers) are by default the same ones used to manage TMD symptoms and other TMD-associated comorbidities. The TMD clinician may want to consider ancillary diagnostic modalities including serologic testing in the work-up of the comorbidities that may underlie TMD and TMD pain.

TMD and migraine share the same nociceptive system, the trigeminal nerve. Once activated, the trigeminal nerve carries its signals through the trigeminocervical complex, converging on the trigeminal nucleus caudalis, the central pathway of pain modulation to the thalamus.[20] People with TMD and migraine are also more prone to develop allodynia, a sign of central sensitization. This can be seen during attacks of migraine and also between migraine attacks. Studies show allodynia is present in 86.9% of comorbid myofascial TMD and migraine, but only in 40% of those with migraine alone.[36] Both diseases may share a similar genetic basis.[21] Headaches that are comorbid with TMD significantly lower the quality of life for these patients. Optimal management of TMD and TMD pain must include diagnosis and appropriate management of the comorbid headache entities.

LOWER BACK PAIN

There is an abundance of literature showing significant association between LBP and TMDs.[37–41] Lower back pain (LBP) has been shown to have higher risk of association with TMDs, and considered a contributing factor in the onset of TMD.[37] Some recent articles have placed a high association between TMD and LBP.[9] Approximately two-thirds of TMD patients reported LBP in a recent large cohort study.[37,38] Other articles have described LBP as a comorbidity with musculoskeletal disorders of the face and jaw.[37,41] Recent study also reported that when LBP became chronic, TMD symptoms became more clinically positive.[37] A prospective study found a greater prevalence of TMD in patients with history of LBP (approximately 50%), compared to subjects with no such history.[42] Considerable overlap of symptoms were found with fibromyalgia, TMD, and LBP.[9] The TMD clinician must ask the patient about pain elsewhere in the body, specifically LBP.

MYOFASCIAL PAIN

Association of pain outside the head and face with TMD and TMD-associated pain has been shown in the early pain literature.[43] Masticatory muscle disorders (MMDs) have been found to be the most prevalent (approximately 45%) in the TMD population, as opposed to much lesser prevalence of the same in the general population (approximately 10%).[44,45] According to the Research Diagnostic Criteria for Temporomandibular Disorders (RDC-TMD)/Diagnostic Criteria for Temporomandibular Disorders (DC-TMD), myofascial pain with referral is subclassified under "myogenous TMD."[46,47] Serologic testing has been suggested in an attempt to delineate the comorbidities that exist with TMDs.[44] A high prevalence of myofascial syndrome was found in patients diagnosed with TMD.[3]

ANXIETY AND DEPRESSION

The association between TMD and such psychological comorbidities as anxiety and depression is well documented in the recent literature.[48–51] The National Institute of

Neurologic Disorders and Stroke (NINDS) has classified TMD under "chronic overlapping pain conditions."[52] Another psychological entity that is comorbid with TMD is post-traumatic stress disorder (PTSD).[53] The recent literature of these associated comorbidities is so robust that it prompted inclusion of psychosocial factors to predict TMD incidence, and to identify TMD subgroups as per psychosocial and biological characteristics.[48,54] In musculoskeletal disorders such as TMD, there is an increased level of proinflammatory cytokines, which, in turn, has correlation with depression and stress.[52,55] TMD and psychological factors as comorbid conditions in children and adolescents have been a subject of discussion in the recent literature,[56–60] with a trend toward higher anxiety and depression in this population.[61] A mechanistic explanation of the association of depression and anxiety as comorbidities of TMDs is only evolving in the current literature. The role of neurotransmitters common to pain and depression has been proposed. Serotonin, and its role in TMDs, depression, and central and peripheral sensitizations, has been seen as one of the possible mechanisms of this association.[62,63] Another plausible explanation is genetic association between TMDs, depression and anxiety. Systemic inflammation involving a higher level of proinflammatory cytokines has been proposed to have an effect on neurotransmitter systems, thereby bringing about such behavioral changes as anhedonia, anxiety, and depression.[64] The same literature has also shown that these proinflammatory agents adversely affect the synthesis and function of monoamines such as serotonin, dopamine, and norepinephrine. Consequently, a management program that may consistently target and reduce systemic inflammation may in turn be more beneficial for optimal pain management for TMD patients. This has led to the popular proposal of using NSAIDs for the management of TMDs with concomitant depression and anxiety. The clinician attempting to manage TMD pain must be aware of the strong association of TMD with comorbid psychological conditions such as anxiety and depression, and make the appropriate referrals for effective optimal pain management.

FIBROMYALGIA

Fibromyalgia (FM) has been traditionally seen in the literature as a poster child for central sensitization pain syndromes. Orofacial pain in general, and TMD in particular, have been known to be of high prevalence in FM subjects.[9,65–68] The reported association of FM with TMDs was more with the younger group of patients; older age was found to be more associated with LBP.[9,37] Other recent studies have shown a strong independent association of TMD with FM and other chronic pain syndromes.[4] Studies have shown an approximately 3 to 5 times greater prevalence of FM in TMD patients compared with the general population.[3,69–71] The pharmacologic therapy for FM is similar to that of TMD-associated pain as to the drug classes used. Dysregulation of adrenergic function has been shown in FM and TMD, with altered catecholamine levels compared with normal controls.[72] These findings have led to the use of beta blockers such as propranolol in low doses for management of FM and TMDs. Also to be noted is the use of low doses of antidepressants for the management of FM, comorbid depression, and TMDs.

IRRITABLE BOWEL SYNDROME

Chronic TMD is considered among functional pain syndromes including FM, IBS, and chronic fatigue syndrome (CFS). This is even more true of myofascial TMD.[73,74] There have been several studies associating IBS with TMDs.[75] In a large cohort of a wide age range (18–65 years) of patients with IBS, the risk of having TMD was more than 3 times that of a healthy control group.[76] One study had reported a weak association between

TMD and IBS.[77] A greater risk of IBS has also been shown in TMD patients, and also was observed a more severe form of IBS in TMD patients, compared with healthy controls.[75] Somatic and depressive symptoms were found to be more prevalent with TMD and IBS.[78] Reduced descending/endogenous pain modulation was found in IBS and TMD patients.[79] In view of the mounting evidence of association between IBS and TMD, the treating physician should include a history and/or symptoms of IBS in TMD patients with a higher suspicion of IBS.

CHRONIC FATIGUE SYNDROME

CFS has been shown to be associated with increased intensity and duration of TMD pain.[13] TMD patients presenting with myofascial pain have higher prevalence of self-reported CFS, than those with nonmyofascial TMD.[80] TMD has been shown to not only coexist with CFS and FM, but to share symptomatology also. There is increasing evidence that these three, and other entities, may have similar pathophysiologic mechanisms.[74] A recent systematic review exploring TMD and CFS as comorbidities suggested a potential high overlap between the 2 conditions, stressing the need for rigorous studies for assessment of this relationship.[81]

STOMACH PAIN

One of the interesting TMD pain associations the authors found was stomach pain. Multiple studies spanning across age, gender, and ethnicity showed an association of TMD pain and stomach pain.[82,83] However, some studies have shown negligible[84] or weak[85] association between the 2 entities. Frequent stomach pain was related to long-term TMD, and it was the only comorbidity considerably more frequent in long-term TMD patients compared with short-term TMD patients.[86] An association of TMD pain, preterm birth, and stomach pain was also shown.[82] In a large cohort of stomach pain patients with age ranges 25 to 75, approximately 60% reported occasional TMD pain, and 57% reported having chronic TMD pain.[87] The clinician managing TMD and TMD pain, once again, needs to enquire about other bodily pains including stomach pain.

VULVODYNIA

Orofacial pain conditions including TMD was found to be common in women with vulvodynia and vestibulodynia,[88] leading to the suggestion that there may be common mechanisms mediating these conditions.[89] Other studies on women with vulvodynia showed moderate to strong association of TMD with this entity, as well as other comorbid conditions such as FM and IBS.[90–92]

SLEEP DISORDERS

Sleep disorders including insomnia, obstructive sleep apnea (OSA), and sleep-related bruxism (SRB), have been explored for associations with TMD and TMD pain. A long-term large cohort study recently showed that primary sleep disorders are independent risk factors for both in the initiation and in the maintenance of TMD and TMD pain.[93] Approximately 90% of TMD patients have been shown to have some comorbid sleep disorders.[94–96] The prevalence of TMD has been proposed to be higher in patients with OSA compared with the general population.[97,98] This same literature also shows that TMD-related pain, craniofacial pain, and extraoral pain, show higher prevalence in OSA patients. Further, OSA is considered a comorbidity for TMD and craniofacial pain.[97] OSA has further been shown to be associated with chronic pain disorders including TMD.[99,100] OSA patients have been shown to be more likely to present first-onset TMD.[94,99] The spectrum of TMD as associated with sleep disorders, CFS, and FM has also been proposed.[74] Poor sleep quality is reported in most TMD patients.[93,96,101] There is mounting evidence of sleep disturbances acting as an etiologic factor in the development and pathogenesis of TMDs.[80,93,102]

Insomnia has shown to be of a high prevalence in chronic pain,[103,104] and changes in insomnia symptom and severity are associated with similar changes in the pain experience of the TMD patient.[103] Further, insomnia and related short sleep duration have been shown to be associated with more severe clinical TMD pain profile.[105]

MANAGEMENT OF TEMPOROMANDIBULAR JOINT DISORDERS WITH COMORBIDITIES

Comorbidities should be addressed in an attempt to manage TMD and TMD-related pain. TMD patients should be evaluated for headaches in general, and migraine and TTH in particular.[106] A recently published randomized controlled trial study showed the efficacy of propranolol in reducing TMD pain to be more in migraine sufferers than in nonmigraine sufferers, and the mechanism of this was reduction in the heart rate.[107] The European Alliance of Associations for Rheumatology (EULAR) guidelines recommend the use of nonpharmacological treatment for central sensitization syndromes such as FM.[108] There are also several management modalities that have also shown efficacy in TMD and TMD pain.[109] Biofeedback and cognitive behavioral therapies (CBT) have been shown to improve coping skills in TMD pain and are well accepted by patients.[110] Other studies have shown that CBT and biofeedback employing surface electromyographic training of the masticatory muscles are also efficacious in TMD pain management.[111] On the contrary, a systematic review had shown that there is insufficient evidence to firmly recommend the use of CBT in the management of TMD.[112] However, when CBT was combined with pharmacologic therapy, it yielded superior results in pain reduction, improvement of depression, and improvement of quality of life in chronic TMD patients.[113] Pharmacologically, TMD and TMD pain are managed with several classes of medications including, but not limited to NSAIDs, steroids, skeletal muscle relaxants, antidepressants, and anticonvulsants.[114] The comorbidities that are discussed in this article should be managed using a multidisciplinary referral method for optimal TMD pain management.[115,116] Alternative health care modalities such as acupuncture have shown modest to good efficacy in managing TMD pain.[115,117,118]

CLINICAL PEARLS

Several comorbidities have been shown to exist with TMD and TMD pain. These include, but are not limited to headaches, anxiety, depression, IBS, CFS and FM, sleep disorders, vulvodynia, stomach pain, and LBP. The astute clinician attempting to manage TMD and TMD pain must be well versed with the latest in the literature regarding the association and correlation of comorbidities of TMD. Management philosophies that do not take these into consideration may be narrow and insufficient in achieving optimal pain control in TMD patients. It behooves the clinician to screen for these known comorbidities, order succinct laboratory tests, and make prompt referrals to appropriate specialists and pain management physicians, facilitating a holistic, multidisciplinary management approach. This in turn results in efficient pain management for the patient.

REFERENCES

1. Valderas JM, Starfield B, Sibbald B, et al. Defining comorbidity: implications for understanding health and health services. Ann Fam Med 2009;7(4):357–63.
2. Feinstein AR. The pre-therapeutic classification of co-morbidity in chronic disease. J Chronic Dis 1970;23(7):455–68.
3. Kleykamp BA, Ferguson MC, McNicol E, et al. The prevalence of comorbid chronic pain conditions among patients with temporomandibular disorders: A systematic review. J Am Dent Assoc 2022;153(3):241–50.e10.
4. Sharma S, Slade GD, Fillingim RB, et al. Attributes germane to temporomandibular disorders and their associations with five chronic overlapping pain conditions. J Oral Facial Pain Headache 2020;34:s57–72.
5. Contreras EFR, Fernandes G, Ongaro PCJ, et al. Systemic diseases and other painful conditions in patients with temporomandibular disorders and migraine. Braz Oral Res 2018;32:e77.
6. Maixner W, Fillingim RB, Williams DA, et al. Overlapping chronic pain conditions: implications for diagnosis and classification. J Pain 2016;17(9 Suppl):T93–107.
7. Fernandes G, Arruda MA, Bigal ME, et al. Painful temporomandibular disorder is associated with migraine in adolescents: a case-control study. J Pain 2019; 20(10):1155–63.
8. Natoli JL, Manack A, Dean B, et al. Global prevalence of chronic migraine: a systematic review. Cephalalgia 2010;30(5):599–609.
9. Slade GD, Greenspan JD, Fillingim RB, et al. Overlap of five chronic pain conditions: temporomandibular disorders, headache, back pain, irritable bowel syndrome, and fibromyalgia. J Oral Facial Pain Headache 2020;34:s15–28.
10. Franco AL, Gonçalves DA, Castanharo SM, et al. Migraine is the most prevalent primary headache in individuals with temporomandibular disorders. J Orofac Pain 2010;24(3):287–92.
11. Tchivileva IE, Ohrbach R, Fillingim RB, et al. Temporal change in headache and its contribution to the risk of developing first-onset temporomandibular disorder in the Orofacial Pain: Prospective Evaluation and Risk Assessment (OPPERA) study. Pain 2017;158(1):120–9.
12. Svensson P. Muscle pain in the head: overlap between temporomandibular disorders and tension-type headaches. Curr Opin Neurol 2007;20(3):320–5.
13. Dahan H, Shir Y, Velly A, et al. Specific and number of comorbidities are associated with increased levels of temporomandibular pain intensity and duration. J Headache Pain 2015;16:528.
14. Gonçalves DA, Camparis CM, Speciali JG, et al. Temporomandibular disorders are differentially associated with headache diagnoses: a controlled study. Clin J Pain 2011;27(7):611–5.
15. Kang JK, Ryu JW, Choi JH, et al. Application of ICHD-II criteria for headaches in a TMJ and orofacial pain clinic. Cephalalgia 2010;30(1):37–41.
16. Fragoso YD, Alves HH, Garcia SO, et al. Prevalence of parafunctional habits and temporomandibular dysfunction symptoms in patients attending a tertiary headache clinic. Arq Neuropsiquiatr 2010;68(3):377–80.
17. da Silva A Jr, Costa EC, Gomes JB, et al. Chronic headache and comorbidities: a two-phase, population-based, cross-sectional study. Headache 2010;50(8): 1306–12.
18. Ballegaard V, Thede-Schmidt-Hansen P, Svensson P, et al. Are headache and temporomandibular disorders related? A blinded study. Cephalalgia 2008; 28(8):832–41.

19. Mitrirattanakul S, Merrill RL. Headache impact in patients with orofacial pain. J Am Dent Assoc 2006;137(9):1267–74.
20. Graff-Radford SB, Abbott JJ. Temporomandibular disorders and headache. Oral Maxillofacial Surg Clin N Am 2016;28(3):335–49.
21. Speciali JG, Dach F. Temporomandibular dysfunction and headache disorder. Headache 2015;55(Suppl 1):72–83.
22. Shu H, Liu S, Tang Y, et al. A pre-existing myogenic temporomandibular disorder increases trigeminal calcitonin gene-related peptide and enhances nitroglycerin-induced hypersensitivity in mice. Int J Mol Sci 2020;21(11). https://doi.org/10.3390/ijms21114049.
23. Anderson GC, John MT, Ohrbach R, et al. Influence of headache frequency on clinical signs and symptoms of TMD in subjects with temple headache and TMD pain. Pain 2011;152(4):765–71.
24. Bevilaqua Grossi D, Lipton RB, Bigal ME. Temporomandibular disorders and migraine chronification. Curr Pain Headache Rep 2009;13(4):314–8.
25. Fernandes G, Franco AL, Gonçalves DA, et al. Temporomandibular disorders, sleep bruxism, and primary headaches are mutually associated. J Orofac Pain 2013;27(1):14–20.
26. Headache Classification Committee of the International Headache Society (IHS) The International Classification of Headache Disorders. Cephalalgia 2018;38(1): 1–211, 3rd edition.
27. Conti PC, Costa YM, Gonçalves DA, et al. Headaches and myofascial temporo-mandibular disorders: overlapping entities, separate managements? J Oral Rehabil 2016;43(9):702–15.
28. Lim PF, Smith S, Bhalang K, et al. Development of temporomandibular disorders is associated with greater bodily pain experience. Clin J Pain 2010;26(2): 116–20.
29. LeResche L, Mancl LA, Drangsholt MT, et al. Predictors of onset of facial pain and temporomandibular disorders in early adolescence. Pain 2007;129(3): 269–78.
30. Von Korff M, Resche LL, Dworkin SF. First onset of common pain symptoms: a prospective study of depression as a risk factor. Pain 1993;55(2):251–8.
31. Yakkaphan P, Smith JG, Chana P, et al. Temporomandibular disorder and head-ache prevalence: a systematic review and meta-analysis. Cephalalgia Rep 2022;5. 25158163221097352.
32. Michelotti A, de Wijer A, Steenks M, et al. Home-exercise regimes for the man-agement of non-specific temporomandibular disorders. J Oral Rehabil 2005; 32(11):779–85.
33. Medlicott MS, Harris SR. A systematic review of the effectiveness of exercise, manual therapy, electrotherapy, relaxation training, and biofeedback in the man-agement of temporomandibular disorder. Phys Ther 2006;86(7):955–73.
34. Fricton J, Look JO, Wright E, et al. Systematic review and meta-analysis of ran-domized controlled trials evaluating intraoral orthopedic appliances for tempo-romandibular disorders. J Orofac Pain 2010;24(3):237–54.
35. Gatchel RJ, Stowell AW, Wildenstein L, et al. Efficacy of an early intervention for patients with acute temporomandibular disorder-related pain: a one-year outcome study. J Am Dent Assoc 2006;137(3):339–47.
36. Bevilaqua-Grossi D, Lipton RB, Napchan U, et al. Temporomandibular disorders and cutaneous allodynia are associated in individuals with migraine. Cephalal-gia 2010;30(4):425–32.

37. Lee KC, Wu YT, Chien WC, et al. The prevalence of first-onset temporomandibular disorder in low back pain and associated risk factors: A nationwide population-based cohort study with a 15-year follow-up. Medicine (Baltimore) 2020;99(3):e18686.

38. Plesh O, Adams SH, Gansky SA. Temporomandibular joint and muscle disorder-type pain and comorbid pains in a national US sample. J Orofac Pain 2011; 25(3):190–8.

39. Sipilä K, Suominen AL, Alanen P, et al. Association of clinical findings of temporomandibular disorders (TMD) with self-reported musculoskeletal pains. Eur J Pain 2011;15(10):1061–7.

40. Wiesinger B, Malker H, Englund E, et al. Does a dose-response relation exist between spinal pain and temporomandibular disorders? BMC Musculoskelet Disord 2009;10:28.

41. Wiesinger B, Malker H, Englund E, et al. Back pain in relation to musculoskeletal disorders in the jaw-face: a matched case-control study. Pain 2007;131(3): 311–9.

42. Sanders AE, Slade GD, Bair E, et al. General health status and incidence of first-onset temporomandibular disorder: the OPPERA prospective cohort study. J Pain 2013;14(12 Suppl):T51–62.

43. Türp JC, Kowalski CJ, Stohler CS. Temporomandibular disorders–pain outside the head and face is rarely acknowledged in the chief complaint. J Prosthet Dent 1997;78(6):592–5.

44. Kalladka M, Young A, Khan J. Myofascial pain in temporomandibular disorders: Updates on etiopathogenesis and management. J Bodyw Mov Ther 2021;28: 104–13.

45. Manfredini D, Guarda-Nardini L, Winocur E, et al. Research diagnostic criteria for temporomandibular disorders: a systematic review of axis I epidemiologic findings. Oral Surg Oral Med Oral Pathol Oral Radiol Endod 2011;112(4): 453–62.

46. Barjandi G, Kosek E, Hedenberg-Magnusson B, et al. Comorbid conditions in temporomandibular disorders myalgia and myofascial pain compared to fibromyalgia. J Clin Med 2021;10(14). https://doi.org/10.3390/jcm10143138.

47. Schiffman E, Ohrbach R, Truelove E, et al. Diagnostic criteria for temporomandibular disorders (DC/TMD) for clinical and research applications: recommendations of the International RDC/TMD Consortium Network* and Orofacial Pain Special Interest Group†. J Oral Facial Pain Headache 2014;28(1):6–27.

48. Lira MR, Lemes da Silva RR, Bataglion C, et al. Multiple diagnoses, increased kinesiophobia? - Patients with high kinesiophobia levels showed a greater number of temporomandibular disorder diagnoses. Musculoskelet Sci Pract 2019; 44:102054.

49. Kothari SF, Baad-Hansen L, Svensson P. Psychosocial profiles of temporomandibular disorder pain patients: proposal of a new approach to present complex data. J Oral Facial Pain Headache 2017;31(3):199–209.

50. Bertoli E, de Leeuw R. Prevalence of suicidal ideation, depression, and anxiety in chronic temporomandibular disorder patients. J Oral Facial Pain Headache 2016;30(4):296–301.

51. Reiter S, Emodi-Perlman A, Goldsmith C, et al. Comorbidity between depression and anxiety in patients with temporomandibular disorders according to the research diagnostic criteria for temporomandibular disorders. J Oral Facial Pain Headache 2015;29(2):135–43.

52. Fenton BT, Goulet JL, Bair MJ, et al. Relationships between temporomandibular disorders, MSD conditions, and mental health comorbidities: findings from the Veterans Musculoskeletal Disorders Cohort. Pain Med 2018;19(suppl_1):S61–8.

53. Mottaghi A, Zamani E. Temporomandibular joint health status in war veterans with post-traumatic stress disorder. J Educ Health Promot 2014;3:60.

54. Slade GD, Ohrbach R, Greenspan JD, et al. Painful temporomandibular disorder: decade of discovery from OPPERA studies. J Dent Res 2016;95(10): 1084–92.

55. Zorina-Lichtenwalter K, Meloto CB, Khoury S, et al. Genetic predictors of human chronic pain conditions. Neuroscience 2016;338:36–62.

56. Sangalli L, Gibler R, Boggero I. Pediatric chronic orofacial pain: a narrative review of biopsychosocial associations and treatment approaches. Front Pain Res (Lausanne) 2021;2:790420.

57. de Paiva Bertoli FM, Bruzamolin CD, de Almeida Kranz GO, et al. Anxiety and malocclusion are associated with temporomandibular disorders in adolescents diagnosed by RDC/TMD. A cross-sectional study. J Oral Rehabil 2018;45(10): 747–55.

58. Kobayashi FY, Gavião MBD, Marquezin MCS, et al. Salivary stress biomarkers and anxiety symptoms in children with and without temporomandibular disorders. Braz Oral Res 2017;31:e78.

59. Nilsson IM, Drangsholt M, List T. Impact of temporomandibular disorder pain in adolescents: differences by age and gender. J Orofac Pain 2009;23(2):115–22.

60. Wahlund K, List T, Ohrbach R. The relationship between somatic and emotional stimuli: a comparison between adolescents with temporomandibular disorders (TMD) and a control group. Eur J Pain 2005;9(2):219–27.

61. Al-Khotani A, Naimi-Akbar A, Gjelset M, et al. The associations between psychosocial aspects and TMD-pain related aspects in children and adolescents. J Headache Pain 2016;17:30.

62. Shrivastava M, Battaglino R, Ye L. A comprehensive review on biomarkers associated with painful temporomandibular disorders. Int J Oral Sci 2021;13(1):23.

63. Ernberg M, Voog U, Alstergren P, et al. Plasma and serum serotonin levels and their relationship to orofacial pain and anxiety in fibromyalgia. J Orofac Pain 2000;14(1):37–46.

64. Miller AH, Raison CL. The role of inflammation in depression: from evolutionary imperative to modern treatment target. Nat Rev Immunol 2016;16(1):22–34.

65. Ayouni I, Chebbi R, Hela Z, et al. Comorbidity between fibromyalgia and temporomandibular disorders: a systematic review. Oral Surg Oral Med Oral Pathol Oral Radiol 2019;128(1):33–42.

66. Wolfe F, Clauw DJ, Fitzcharles MA, et al. The American College of Rheumatology preliminary diagnostic criteria for fibromyalgia and measurement of symptom severity. Arthritis Care Res (Hoboken) 2010;62(5):600–10.

67. Balasubramaniam R, de Leeuw R, Zhu H, et al. Prevalence of temporomandibular disorders in fibromyalgia and failed back syndrome patients: a blinded prospective comparison study. Oral Surg Oral Med Oral Pathol Oral Radiol Endod 2007;104(2):204–16.

68. Leblebici B, Pektaş ZO, Ortancil O, et al. Coexistence of fibromyalgia, temporomandibular disorder, and masticatory myofascial pain syndromes. Rheumatol Int 2007;27(6):541–4.

69. Jones GT, Atzeni F, Beasley M, et al. The prevalence of fibromyalgia in the general population: a comparison of the American College of Rheumatology 1990,

2010, and modified 2010 classification criteria. Arthritis Rheumatol 2015;67(2): 568–75.

70. Branco JC, Bannwarth B, Failde I, et al. Prevalence of fibromyalgia: a survey in five European countries. Semin Arthritis Rheum 2010;39(6):448–53.

71. Neumann L, Buskila D. Epidemiology of fibromyalgia. Curr Pain Headache Rep 2003;7(5):362–8.

72. Light KC, Bragdon EE, Grewen KM, et al. Adrenergic dysregulation and pain with and without acute beta-blockade in women with fibromyalgia and temporomandibular disorder. J Pain 2009;10(5):542–52.

73. Furquim BD, Flamengui LM, Conti PC. TMD and chronic pain: a current view. Dental Press J Orthod 2015;20(1):127–33.

74. Aaron LA, Burke MM, Buchwald D. Overlapping conditions among patients with chronic fatigue syndrome, fibromyalgia, and temporomandibular disorder. Arch Intern Med 2000;160(2):221–7.

75. Mobilio N, Iovino P, Bruno V, et al. Severity of irritable bowel syndrome in patients with temporomandibular disorders: a case-control study. J Clin Exp Dent 2019; 11(9):e802–6.

76. Gallotta S, Bruno V, Catapano S, et al. High risk of temporomandibular disorder in irritable bowel syndrome: Is there a correlation with greater illness severity? World J Gastroenterol 2017;23(1):103–9.

77. Burris JL, Evans DR, Carlson CR. Psychological correlates of medical comorbidities in patients with temporomandibular disorders. J Am Dent Assoc 2010; 141(1):22–31.

78. Sanders AE, Weatherspoon ED, Ehrmann BM, et al. Ratio of omega-6/omega-3 polyunsaturated fatty acids associated with somatic and depressive symptoms in people with painful temporomandibular disorder and irritable bowel syndrome. J Pain 2022. https://doi.org/10.1016/j.jpain.2022.04.006.

79. King CD, Wong F, Currie T, et al. Deficiency in endogenous modulation of prolonged heat pain in patients with irritable bowel syndrome and temporomandibular disorder. Pain 2009;143(3):172–8.

80. Dahan H, Shir Y, Nicolau B, et al. Self-reported migraine and chronic fatigue syndrome are more prevalent in people with myofascial vs nonmyofascial temporomandibular disorders. J Oral Facial Pain Headache 2016;30(1):7–13.

81. Robinson LJ, Durham J, Newton JL. A systematic review of the comorbidity between temporomandibular disorders and chronic fatigue syndrome. J Oral Rehabil 2016;43(4):306–16.

82. Nilsson IM, Brogårdh-Roth S, Månsson J, et al. Temporomandibular pain in adolescents with a history of preterm birth. J Oral Rehabil 2019;46(7):589–96.

83. Al-Harthy M, Michelotti A, List T, et al. Influence of culture on pain comorbidity in women with and without temporomandibular disorder-pain. J Oral Rehabil 2017; 44(6):415–25.

84. Nilsson IM, List T, Drangsholt M. Headache and co-morbid pains associated with TMD pain in adolescents. J Dent Res 2013;92(9):802–7.

85. Khan K, Muller-Bolla M, Anacleto Teixeira Junior O, et al. Comorbid conditions associated with painful temporomandibular disorders in adolescents from Brazil, Canada and France: a cross-sectional study. J Oral Rehabil 2020; 47(4):417–24.

86. Velly AM, Botros J, Bolla MM, et al. Painful and non-painful comorbidities associated with short- and long-term painful temporomandibular disorders: a cross-sectional study among adolescents from Brazil, Canada and France. J Oral Rehabil 2022;49(3):273–82.

87. Visscher CM, Ligthart L, Schuller AA, et al. Comorbid disorders and sociodemographic variables in temporomandibular pain in the general Dutch population. J Oral Facial Pain Headache 2015;29(1):51–9.

88. Zolnoun DA, Rohl J, Moore CG, et al. Overlap between orofacial pain and vulvar vestibulitis syndrome. Clin J Pain 2008;24(3):187–91.

89. Bair E, Simmons E, Hartung J, et al. Natural history of comorbid orofacial pain among women with vestibulodynia. Clin J Pain 2015;31(1):73–8.

90. Nguyen RH, Veasley C, Smolenski D. Latent class analysis of comorbidity patterns among women with generalized and localized vulvodynia: preliminary findings. J Pain Res 2013;6:303–9.

91. Nguyen RH, Ecklund AM, Maclehose RF, et al. Co-morbid pain conditions and feelings of invalidation and isolation among women with vulvodynia. Psychol Health Med 2012;17(5):589–98.

92. Arnold LD, Bachmann GA, Rosen R, et al. Assessment of vulvodynia symptoms in a sample of US women: a prevalence survey with a nested case control study. Am J Obstet Gynecol 2007;196(2):128.e1–6.

93. Kim SJ, Park SM, Cho HJ, et al. The relationship between primary sleep disorders and temporomandibular disorders: an 8-year nationwide cohort study in South Korea. Int J Gen Med 2021;14:7121–31.

94. Alessandri-Bonetti A, Scarano E, Fiorita A, et al. Prevalence of signs and symptoms of temporo-mandibular disorder in patients with sleep apnea. Sleep Breath 2021;25(4):2001–6.

95. Sener S, Guler O. Self-reported data on sleep quality and psychologic characteristics in patients with myofascial pain and disc displacement versus asymptomatic controls. Int J Prosthodont 2012;25(4):348–52.

96. Rener-Sitar K, John MT, Pusalavidyasagar SS, et al. Sleep quality in temporomandibular disorder cases. Sleep Med 2016;25:105–12.

97. Spencer J, Patel M, Mehta N, et al. Special consideration regarding the assessment and management of patients being treated with mandibular advancement oral appliance therapy for snoring and obstructive sleep apnea. Cranio 2013; 31(1):10–3.

98. Cunali PA, Almeida FR, Santos CD, et al. Prevalence of temporomandibular disorders in obstructive sleep apnea patients referred for oral appliance therapy. J Orofac Pain 2009;23(4):339–44.

99. Sanders AE, Essick GK, Fillingim R, et al. Sleep apnea symptoms and risk of temporomandibular disorder: OPPERA cohort. J Dent Res 2013;92(7 Suppl): 70s–7s.

100. Smith MT, Wickwire EM, Grace EG, et al. Sleep disorders and their association with laboratory pain sensitivity in temporomandibular joint disorder. Sleep 2009; 32(6):779–90.

101. Yatani H, Studts J, Cordova M, et al. Comparison of sleep quality and clinical and psychologic characteristics in patients with temporomandibular disorders. J Orofac Pain 2002;16(3):221–8.

102. Sanders AE, Akinkugbe AA, Fillingim RB, et al. Causal mediation in the development of painful temporomandibular disorder. J Pain 2017;18(4):428–36.

103. Quartana PJ, Wickwire EM, Klick B, et al. Naturalistic changes in insomnia symptoms and pain in temporomandibular joint disorder: a cross-lagged panel analysis. Pain 2010;149(2):325–31.

104. Abad VC, Sarinas PS, Guilleminault C. Sleep and rheumatologic disorders. Sleep Med Rev 2008;12(3):211–28.

105. Lerman SF, Mun CJ, Hunt CA, et al. Insomnia with objective short sleep duration in women with temporomandibular joint disorder: quantitative sensory testing, inflammation and clinical pain profiles. Sleep Med 2022;90:26–35.
106. Tchivileva IE, Hadgraft H, Lim PF, et al. Efficacy and safety of propranolol for treatment of temporomandibular disorder pain: a randomized, placebo-controlled clinical trial. Pain 2020;161(8):1755–67.
107. Tchivileva IE, Ohrbach R, Fillingim RB, et al. Effect of comorbid migraine on propranolol efficacy for painful TMD in a randomized controlled trial. Cephalalgia 2021;41(7):839–50.
108. Macfarlane GJ, Kronisch C, Dean LE, et al. EULAR revised recommendations for the management of fibromyalgia. Ann Rheum Dis 2017;76(2):318–28.
109. Atzeni F, Talotta R, Masala IF, et al. One year in review 2019: fibromyalgia. Clin Exp Rheumatol 2019;37(Suppl 116):3–10.
110. Shedden Mora MC, Weber D, Neff A, et al. Biofeedback-based cognitive-behavioral treatment compared with occlusal splint for temporomandibular disorder: a randomized controlled trial. Clin J Pain 2013;29(12):1057–65.
111. Crider A, Glaros AG, Gevirtz RN. Efficacy of biofeedback-based treatments for temporomandibular disorders. Appl Psychophysiol Biofeedback 2005;30(4):333–45.
112. Liu HX, Liang QJ, Xiao P, et al. The effectiveness of cognitive-behavioural therapy for temporomandibular disorders: a systematic review. J Oral Rehabil 2012;39(1):55–62.
113. Calderon Pdos S, Tabaquim Mde L, Oliveira LC, et al. Effectiveness of cognitive-behavioral therapy and amitriptyline in patients with chronic temporomandibular disorders: a pilot study. Braz Dent J 2011;22(5):415–21.
114. Ouanounou A, Goldberg M, Haas DA. Pharmacotherapy in temporomandibular disorders: a review. J Can Dent Assoc 2017;83:h7.
115. Kapos FP, Exposto FG, Oyarzo JF, et al. Temporomandibular disorders: a review of current concepts in aetiology, diagnosis and management. Oral Surg 2020;13(4):321–34.
116. Haviv Y, Rettman A, Aframian D, et al. Myofascial pain: an open study on the pharmacotherapeutic response to stepped treatment with tricyclic antidepressants and gabapentin. J Oral Facial Pain Headache 2015;29(2):144–51.
117. Fernandes AC, Duarte Moura DM, Da Silva LGD, et al. Acupuncture in Temporomandibular Disorder Myofascial Pain Treatment: A Systematic Review. J Oral Facial Pain Headache 2017;31(3):225–32.
118. Yuan QL, Wang P, Liu L, et al. Acupuncture for musculoskeletal pain: A meta-analysis and meta-regression of sham-controlled randomized clinical trials. Sci Rep 2016;6:30675.

Moving?

Make sure your subscription moves with you!

To notify us of your new address, find your **Clinics Account Number** (located on your mailing label above your name), and contact customer service at:

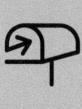

Email: journalscustomerservice-usa@elsevier.com

800-654-2452 (subscribers in the U.S. & Canada)
314-447-8871 (subscribers outside of the U.S. & Canada)

Fax number: 314-447-8029

Elsevier Health Sciences Division
Subscription Customer Service
3251 Riverport Lane
Maryland Heights, MO 63043

*To ensure uninterrupted delivery of your subscription, please notify us at least 4 weeks in advance of move.

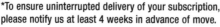

Printed and bound by CPI Group (UK) Ltd, Croydon, CR0 4YY

03/10/2024

01040469-0001